it's just our new normal

normal

from a diagnosis of cystic fibrosis to life

it's just our new normal

from a diagnosis of cystic fibrosis to life

Grace McKenzie

A catalogue record for this book is available from the British Library.

Published by Kindle Direct Publishing

ISBN: 9781717917447

'Remember that hope is a good thing, maybe the best of things, and no good thing ever dies.'

- Rita Hayworth and Shawshank Redemption, Stephen King

Before there was you,
I just never knew.
But,
baba,
you came true
and now
it's all about you.

Dedicated to our beautiful little son. This is for
you, my friend.
May it bring warmth and hope to you and all
those in our situation. Keep smiling and enjoy
your game of life!

Prologue

Some time before you came to meet us, like many expectant parents, we watched several episodes of *One Born Every Minute*. I remember only two people from all of them – a lady in her 40's having her first child, and a lovely, curly haired brunette having a third child to add to her young family.

I guess I remember the lady in her 40's because, I too, was going to be an 'older' first time mother. I have no idea why the other lady stuck so vividly in my mind; even to this day I can see her happy, excited, smiling face and wonder why she in particular settled herself so profoundly in my mind. Her story? Well, she had cystic fibrosis.

Was it a sign from the future, a warning? Or a gentle reassurance that it's all going to be ok cos look at her: she's happy, healthy and having babies. Is that why I always had her in my mind? Cystic fibrosis could not have been further from my awareness. After all, why would it be on my radar? It should've been no different to any of the other stories: watched then forgotten. To this day, I am in awe - knowing what we know now - of her story always having stayed with me. Seems a bit weird, but then again, believing in the weird (and wonderful) may just be part of what keeps our family sane.

Telly off, I carried you within me and continued about my business, smiling as I thought about when it would be our turn to meet our little bundle of joy.

Completely oblivious to what lay ahead.

Welcome to our World

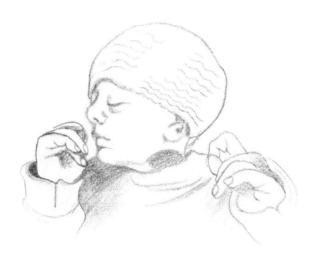

Your daddy and I both waited a long time for you. I was in my late thirties when we got married and we'd already been trying for the best part of a year. Obviously, we were going to struggle. I started to think I'd left it too late. When I did realise I was pregnant, we were both overjoyed. Excited, surprised, shocked even. Age aside, you were a straight forward pregnancy, with only a short spell of nausea (could barely even refer to it as morning sickness!), no high blood pressure and no other issues. The only thing that actually blighted the experience slightly, was that by the last six weeks or so, I developed crippling pains that started at my left foot, shifted to my knee then rode up to my thigh and hip and set up camp. By your due date, I was completely reliant on a walking stick. To my horror, this was to only get worse and would end with us leaving hospital with our sweet new baby, me on crutches. (Not merrily skipping out with you safely tucked in your car seat, heading towards Dobbies for a celebratory coffee and chips, as I'd planned).

Oh, you were the most beautiful baby we had ever seen! I know we are biased, but just look at your photos and tell me you aren't absolutely stunning – like a perfect doll. I could actually not believe that *we* made *you*. Way out of our league (well, mine. Daddy has the looks)!

Not only the hip pain, but there had been a complication with my bladder and I had had to spend 48 hours in bed with a catheter. I could hardly move in the bed with my hip and leg pain, let alone get up and shoogle you in my arms like I longed to do. I longed to just feel like any other new mother – normal. None of that part panned out as I'd envisaged. Sod, and after such a smooth pregnancy; that's what you get for feeling smug, I guess. I *was* able to start the breastfeeding process though (the less said about the first few weeks of *that*, the better), so that gave me some sense of accomplishment and normality at least. Ugh, I was certainly looking forward to getting home and praying for a speedy recovery so I could push you proudly in your pram.

Notably, I remember the car bouncing over speed bumps as we drove from the hospital, two days after giving birth, saying something along the lines of 'Thank God we're getting the hell out of there! Bye-bye hospital!' Little did we know how soon we'd have to come back. And under such polar opposite states of mind.

Aches and pains aside, bringing you home was as confusing and scary as it was exciting and exhilarating. We were beaming with pride at our beautiful, perfect son. We couldn't believe how gorgeous you were, straight from birth. Everyone was going to be as in love with you as we were. Oh, we felt so in love with you! There's no denying that those early days were hard work and, as new parents, we weren't all that sure of everything we were doing or were meant to be doing, but trusted our instincts. I think one of the benefits of being older, for me anyway, was I didn't freak out as much as I may have in the past. I felt confident enough in my nurturing abilities to do the right thing. I guess having had so many pets in my life and having cared quite intensely for some of them also stood me in decent stead for motherhood. Something I think only those who have cared for animals would understand or accept, but anyway, it's true. No, animals aren't babies, but they do depend on you for so much, in health as well as in sickness.

I couldn't believe the exhaustion from the sleepless nights. It was like a twilight zone or something. Sure, I've been tired before and I've been jetlagged before, but this was in a class of its own. I think I broke a few rules in those early days (probably still am), such as allowing you to fall asleep on me after a feed. Actually, I don't think it was as much 'allowing' you as not having a choice cos by the time you were done I literally couldn't keep my eyes open any longer. At least you never fell off the bed (I almost did, but you stayed put) and I never rolled on top of you – hell, I'd slept with a small cat under the covers with me for long enough and if I'd managed not to squish her, then you were going to be ok.

When you were five days old we took you for your heel prick test. It was another run of the

9

mill test as far as we were concerned; I was more aware of my inability to stand up straight unaided than of much else. It was also our first taste of anything resembling traumatic for you, since birth of course, and it was rather an unpleasant hour for all of us. I was encouraged to try feeding you, which did seem to help you settle. There were two midwives that day, I think one was a student, and to add to the stress of it all they didn't get enough blood to complete the sheet so had to do the whole thing again. When they left the room, mummy and daddy rolled their eyes at each other as we tried to comfort you. Your poor little foot!

We loved dressing you in the adorable baby clothes and every day you got cuter and cuter. The house was a mess with all the new paraphernalia one simply *must have* when they bring a baby into their world, but it didn't matter - it was just a new kind of mess. I'm not going to pretend it was all lullabies and cuddles though, far from it. We were wrung out and wired all at the same time. Daddy was forever heading to the shops for a smaller set of bodysuits, breast pads, more nappies or more water wipes and mummy was hobbling about on noisy crutches. Oh, their squeak annoyed daddy so, and don't even mention the noise they made if they fell – usually bouncing off the loudest bit of furniture we had before clattering onto the laminate (no, it was never the carpet.

Why would it be the carpet? That wouldn't make any noise!)

Yes, those first weeks were hard. A brand new human in the house, every need to be met by us. The sleepless nights, the sweaty, spaced out days with no time or energy to shower or bath, the crippling pain in my leg, the midwife visits (as helpful and well-meaning as they were, they seemed to go on forever), the exhausted evenings trying to fit in physiotherapy on my hip and get a sit-down on a hot water bottle for pain relief. God, I dreaded daddy going back to work, how in the hell was I going to cope, emotionally never mind physically.

The days went on like that and daddy did go back to work. Granny (my mum) came in to help as much as she could. A few weeks later, while you were having a nap, I stood at the window with my hand wrapped around a mug of tea and thought *I guess everything was fine with the heel prick test then, since I haven't heard.* I specifically remember cos it was merely a few hours later on that exact day that I had a missed call and voicemail from the midwives. Something about 'further investigations' regarding the heel prick results.

My head went into a spin. *What are they talking about?* I couldn't even remember what the heel prick was testing for; the midwives had run through the list of conditions or diseases or

11

whatever they were, as if they were an afterthought. And, to us, they may as well have been an afterthought; another box to tick. I grabbed my laptop and thumped 'NHS newborn heel prick test' into Google. I can't lie, I was feeling a little sick.

'Every baby is offered newborn blood spot screening, also known as the heel prick test, ideally when they are five days old. Newborn blood spot screening involves taking a blood sample to find out if your baby has one of nine rare but serious health conditions. Most babies screened won't have any of these conditions but, for the few who do, the benefits of screening are enormous. Early treatment can improve their health, and prevent severe disability or even death. Conditions tested for:

Sickle Cell Disease *- About 1 in 2,000 babies born in the UK has sickle cell disease. This is a serious inherited blood disease. Sickle cell disease affects haemoglobin, the iron-rich protein in red blood cells that carries oxygen around the body. Babies who have this condition will need specialist care throughout their lives. People with sickle cell disease can have attacks of severe pain and get serious, life-threatening infections. They are usually anaemic because their blood cells have difficulty carrying oxygen. The blood spot screening test means that babies with sickle cell disease can receive early treatment to help* *them live healthier lives. This may include vaccinations and antibiotics to prevent serious illnesses. Pregnant women are also routinely tested for sickle cell disease early in pregnancy.*

***Cystic Fibrosis** - About 1 in 2,500 babies born in the UK has cystic fibrosis. This inherited condition affects the digestion and lungs. Babies with cystic fibrosis may not gain weight well and frequently have chest infections. Babies with the condition can be treated early with a high-energy diet, medicines and physiotherapy. Although children with cystic fibrosis may still become very ill, early treatment can help them live longer, healthier lives.*

***Congenital Hypothyroidism** - About 1 in 3,000 babies born in the UK has congenital hypothyroidism. Babies with congenital hypothyroidism do not have enough of the hormone thyroxine. Without thyroxine, babies do not grow properly and can develop learning disabilities. Babies who have the condition can be treated early with thyroxine tablets, and this allows them to develop normally.*

***Inherited metabolic diseases** - It is important to let your health professional know if you have a family history of a metabolic disease (a disease that affects your metabolism). Babies are screened for six inherited metabolic diseases. These are: phenylketonuria (PKU), medium-chain* *acyl-CoA dehydrogenase deficiency (MCADD), maple syrup urine disease (MSUD), isovaleric acidaemia (IVA), glutaric aciduria type 1 (GA1) and homocystinuria (pyridoxine unresponsive) (HCU).*

About 1 in 10,000 babies born in the UK has PKU or MCADD. The other conditions are rarer, occurring in 1 in 100,000 to 150,000 babies. Without treatment, babies with inherited metabolic diseases can become suddenly and seriously ill. The diseases all have different symptoms. Depending on which one affects your baby, the condition may be life-threatening or cause severe developmental problems. They can all be treated with a carefully managed diet and, in some cases, medicines as well. Our bodies break down protein foods like meat and fish into amino acids (the building blocks of protein). Any amino acids that aren't needed are usually broken down and removed from the body. Babies with the inherited metabolic diseases that are screened for are unable to break down one or more amino acids. When levels of these amino acids get very high, they are harmful.'

I had been asked to call a specific number at the hospital, which only added to my alarm. *Why the hospital? What is wrong?* It was all extremely confusing and stressful. That phone call was a bit muddled too; whoever I spoke to didn't have – or couldn't give me – any details at that point, and I would have to call back in a bit.

I got on the phone to the health visitor. No, she hadn't heard anything about it, there was nothing in our notes at their end, and yes she would be informed if anything was wrong. She advised me to try not to worry, it could very well be due to the messed up test and they may just need it redone – it happens, she reassured me.

I was buzzing by now, and not in the good way. Pacing up and down, biting my bottom lip between my teeth, I stared hard at you and wondered how on earth there could be something wrong with such a perfect little thing. *Please God, don't let there be anything wrong with him!*

But when I did call the hospital number back, I heard something that would change everything.

'Hello, you're through to the children's cystic fibrosis nurse. Sorry I can't come to the phone right now, but if you leave your name, number and a short message, I'll get back to you as soon as I can……'

* Beep *

Not a Death Sentence

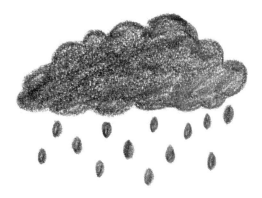

Silence.
Just my shallow breathing.

Cystic fibrosis nurse......?

At first, I thought I'd misheard.
Or maybe I just hoped I had.

WHAT?
No, no, no, no, NO.........!
It was a shock to hear.
It wasn't possible.
It had to be some kind of mistake.

I actually felt the blood drain from my arms.
Nope, that hardly ever happens if you're lucky enough, but it happened right there.
Back onto Google.
Cystic.
Fibrosis.

That's where people have to lie upside down and have their back slapped cos they can't breathe properly, right? But he can't have cystic fibrosis, that's inherited isn't it? And neither of us have it.

In fact, we didn't even know anyone that had it, let alone anyone in our own families. Not that we knew of anyway.

Nah, it can't be that cos we don't have it.
Google had its result.

'Cystic fibrosis is an inherited condition that causes sticky mucus to build up in the lungs and digestive system. This causes lung infections and problems with digesting food. In the UK, most cases of cystic fibrosis are picked up at birth using the newborn screening heel prick test. Symptoms usually start in early childhood and vary from child to child, but the condition gets slowly worse over time, with the lungs and digestive system becoming increasingly damaged. Treatments are available to help reduce the problems caused by the condition and make it easier to live with, but sadly life expectancy is shortened.'

I was silently screaming. *Life expectancy is shortened? WHAT?? You mean, our beautiful new baby is going to die soon?!*

Google continued, *'To be born with cystic fibrosis, a child has to inherit a copy of the faulty gene from both of their parents. This can happen if the parents are "carriers" of the faulty gene, which means they don't have cystic fibrosis themselves. It's estimated around 1 in every 25 people in the UK are carriers of cystic fibrosis.'*

Horror poured into my silently screaming mind. ***We*** *passed it on to him with faulty genes!* I couldn't read anymore. That was enough. I felt a nauseating wave of guilt and grief. *What have we done to our innocent, precious son!*

Haven't we got enough to deal with? I'd thought my leg pain and resulting immobility was bad enough, but just when you think things can't get any worse, something else comes along and shits all over your life.

It seemed unthinkable.
Impossible.

As the tears rolled fast down my cheeks and into my ears, I looked hard at you through blurred eyes. Your beautiful, peaceful face. You were sound asleep in your bouncer, tiny and dwarfed by the colourful prints. You had no idea anything was so wrong. I cried and cried.

After some time, I texted daddy at work and phoned my mum. I had to talk to someone. I said, 'Well I've had some potentially disturbing news.' I had regained some perspective and hope, and almost convinced myself that it wasn't possible and that it must just be that the test needed redone. Life wasn't going to be *that* horrible, right? *We've just brought him home, he can't have this.* Daddy got off work early and we talked for as long as we could bear it.

I re-read the list of conditions the heel prick tested for, and, to be perfectly honest, as awful as cystic fibrosis sounded, it didn't seem to be the absolute worst thing on that list. At least you wouldn't be affected mentally and could live a normal enough life. And it sounded like there were treatments, and the other conditions on the list needed treated too. All-in-all, I didn't feel *quite* so scared and in the dark. I still hoped to God you didn't have it, but, worst case scenario, if it had to be one of those conditions, let it be a treatable one.

It was a full twenty-four hours before I was able to speak to an actual person at the hospital and I can tell you that that was a horribly tense twenty-four hours. All sorts of scenarios ran through our minds. What if it was cystic fibrosis? How were we going to deal with that? We tried not to let our minds go there. It had to be a mistake. They just wanted us to go to the hospital to do the test again, right? (The health visitor had said that if the initial heel prick test was in any way unclear, they would most likely want to re-do it at the hospital nearer the labs cos there is a time limit on these things, a short window to get the right result. Something like that anyway).

When I finally got through, it was all a bit cryptic, in that I shouldn't come to the appointment on my own, could my husband get off work and come with me? And, yes, we did need to come as soon as that, and yes we would be there for a little while. Didn't sound all that positive, but I wasn't ready to give up on the one hope in hell we might still have.

We sat nervously in an in-patient type waiting area. The place was deserted except for someone in reception who headed off down a corridor after taking our names. We waited, rubbing our knuckles and fidgeting our feet. Still hopeful it was just for a re-test.....

As soon as we were led into a room with three people sitting facing us, all hope left. Something was very wrong. We weren't here for anything to be retested; they already *knew*.

No-one spoke.
We sat down.

The biggest man in the room leant forward with folded hands and softly said, 'I'm afraid I have some difficult news for you.'

Oh God! It's one of those rare diseases! He's not going to make it to adulthood!

I was almost relieved when he said you had cystic fibrosis.
But then it all came tumbling down.

Sitting in silence on those seats, we faced a panel of three who now seemed to have some twisted claim on our tiny, precious baby's future. I stared unblinkingly down at you, sound asleep and mercifully oblivious in your car seat. One of them was a doctor, one a nurse and it was unclear who the third was. I hated them already.

As I looked down, to the side, at the doctor, I felt the eyes of the nurse on me and it freaked me out. Perhaps she was ascertaining whether or not we could cope with the news. When I did accidentally catch her eye, she was unsmiling. I wanted to yell *What the hell are you staring at?!*

The doctor rambled on. He had a calm and almost jovial manner. I suppose that was to ease the tension of the situation, not that it did much. I mean, what could make hearing this news about your three week old any easier? Not very much. A good percentage of what he was saying we probably didn't catch, to be fair. We were too stunned and it was too much to take in. *What are they talking about? Why are we here? Why are they talking about this with us? This is all wrong…..this can't be happening to us.*

I wanted to grab you and run from there. I didn't want them to speak about you in this way, to be discussing your future, potential treatments, to touch you or to have anything at all to do with you. I did not want them in my life and I certainly did not want them in your life.

Then another bombshell: he informed us that life expectancy is shortened by cystic fibrosis, but people are living past forty these days. *Forty?! Is that supposed to be **good** news??*

'So, the three of us are all going to die at the same time then?' I blurted out, deliberately trying to sound shocking.

I hoped they were shocked cos I was furious that they were saying this to us. I guess it didn't sink in until later that they would have seen and heard all of these reactions before.

'We know that it's bad news, awful news to hear, but from the point of view of medical advances, there has never been a better time to have cystic fibrosis. Things are changing so fast and the future is much brighter now than it was only a short time ago.' Rambling on, they reassured us that they were there to support us in every way and that you were in the best hands and would be getting the best care.

He went on to explain about the many different variations of the condition, and the variation (or genotype) you had - two copies of DeltaF508 or F508del, the most common one in the UK incidentally, and the one they are currently working on treatments for - and what this meant and how treatment might look. We learnt that both daddy and I were carrying the faulty gene (along with a copy of the 'normal' gene) and had both passed on the faulty copy through no fault of our own; it had been a one in four chance. I felt so guilty, and so sad that we had given this to you.

Confused and anxious, we asked, 'Are we going to find him gasping for air one day?'

'Oh no, no. It's not like that at all.' The nurse assured us.
Well, that's something I suppose.

They went on to explain more of how the symptoms might manifest, such as having to cough up sticky mucus and being more vulnerable to chest infections (caused by bacteria growing in the mucus). The aim of our support team at the hospital was to keep your lungs as healthy as possible for as long as possible; to give you the best start in life. They pointed out how critical the parental role was for your future, how we would become 'experts' on your condition and would be the first port of call for all your cystic fibrosis needs. We were asked many lifestyle questions, such as whether we smoked, how close we were to our families (our support network), how active we were, etc. 'You have a dog? Great! Fresh air and exercise are crucial to those with cystic fibrosis, and, in fact, exercise will become part of your son's physiotherapy programme. No, we've nothing against you living with cats.'

Turned out that you would need daily antibiotics to protect your little lungs from infection, daily physiotherapy (which would start a little later) to clear excess mucus from your lungs, and quite possibly enzymes would have to be added to your every meal to help digest it. First they wanted a poop sample which would be sent to the lab to determine whether or not your pancreatic enzymes were getting through on their own: whether or not you were 'pancreatic insufficient' (meaning you would require the digestive enzymes). It was almost too much to bear. You have to understand, I hardly touched so much as a paracetamol when I was pregnant (until my horrendous leg pain) and it was my intention to raise you as naturally and cleanly as possible, so to hear you would have to start on a daily antibiotic regime was like a blow to the stomach. And the enzymes? 'They're like little hundreds and thousands', (*like that makes it any cuter or easier*) 'and you just sprinkle them onto some apple puree and give with every breastfeed'.

Every breastfeed?
'Yes, every feed.'

Ugh. My instinct was to yell, *No! No. He isn't getting all that poison pumped into his tiny body! For God's sake……he's just a **baby**!*

I suddenly realised that I was thinking about apple puree. I couldn't think where in the hell I could get hold of some.

It became apparent that while we were there, they wanted to get started right away with it all and do some tests and get the medication

27

started. The nurse had her diary out and wanted to give us dates for home visits for herself, the dietician and the physiotherapist. *Oh my God, we're never gonna get rid of these people, are we? They're gonna come to our house, there will be nowhere to hide or get any peace from this! We are never gonna be able to forget and pretend our lives are normal ever again!* I wished we could just get the hell out of there to absorb it. It was a late afternoon in early February, dark and depressing. We felt trapped and confused. They had a good look at you, you were poked and prodded and weighed. You were such a tiny, skinny thing (I remember the doctor saying you had to 'grow into your skin' on the day you were born). I felt so bad waking you up and undressing you in this strange place. The nurse took what she called a 'cough swab' where she basically opened your mouth and stuck a long stick, not dissimilar to a cotton bud, in until you made a coughing sound. This was to check for any bugs in your lungs. *Oh my God, can he have something already?!* Needless to say, you didn't like that very much. And nor did we.

We were left alone momentarily and daddy and I just stared at each other while I breastfed you. Suddenly, he looked at me and mumbled with black humour, 'We can't do anything right.'

By far the worst thing they had to do that afternoon was take bloods from your tiny body.

That was the job of the third person in the seat, who hadn't spoken once. The test was to check the levels of a variety of vital substances within your body, and they were going to take it from your hand. Oh, how you screamed! And how my heart tightened in my chest. I tried to let you suck on my finger to soothe you, but it wasn't hugely successful. The nurse then popped something in your mouth – a glucose substance if I remember right – which is supposed to settle babies under such circumstances. It may or may not have helped a little. I felt my palms sweating and my body weaken under the strain. To see our baby go through so much and to hear you cry so pitifully, was almost too much for mummy and daddy to handle by that point. I held on to you and concentrated on your beautiful face, while we tried to soothe you with our voices and focus on nothing else but you, and for this to be over. A horrendous experience. *It'll be over soon, it'll be over soon.*

Before too long, the nurse returned and took us to a side room for more information overload. We tried to look as composed and accepting as we could, but I felt like I might scream at any moment. I guess the eyes don't lie though, cos the nurse stopped her busying about and looked directly at us, and in such a soft and trusting voice, she said, 'It's not a death sentence.'

At that moment, I believed her (I had to!). She said it with such conviction though, that it brought tears to my eyes and I've never forgotten it to this day. It was one of the few things we'd heard that afternoon that had managed to puncture a tiny enough hole in our bubble of grief to let some of it escape.

She continued, 'He's perfectly healthy at the moment, unaware of any of this. For now, it's your pain, unfortunately.'

I never want it to be your pain, baby. I want to be able to carry it for you forever! I will do my best to keep this pain from you. My head was still reeling that we had passed this on to you.

I wondered about the amount of care you would need and how our lives had suddenly changed completely. It seemed that nothing was going to be simple ever again. The nurse mentioned different benefits that we might be able to claim, and that she would put us in touch with someone who would help us with that side of things. Just more unexpected and unfamiliar news to us. We were told about groups where more experienced parents could offer support to the parents of newly diagnosed children, but we didn't feel that was something we were interested in at that point. I didn't even want to think about it, let alone *talk* about it. We started to think: *We'll definitely need a bigger garden now* and *Will we have to move so we're nearer the hospital?*

Finally, armed with a pile of information leaflets from the Cystic Fibrosis Trust, we were allowed to head home. It was pitch dark and cold outside, mirroring our scattered insides. Once in the car and finally leaving that place (for now; as it turned out, we'd be going back there regularly from then on), I gently turned my head towards daddy and said,

'We *can* do something right. We've made our beautiful, perfect little son.'

We had to gain some perspective! With a heavy and extremely disappointed heart (why couldn't it just have been a bloody botched up heel prick test??), I started texting immediate family with the news. The replies brought with them a little light at the end of a very long, dark tunnel. No-one responded with despair, just plain old common sense and positivity, followed by some researched advice.

Nearly home, daddy stopped off at Tesco for some supplies. God, I wished I could smoke! I'd stopped many years before, but it'd always been my go-to vice in times of stress. Yes, I know, you'd just been diagnosed with a serious lung condition and I was thinking about smoking. How awful of me. But I thought, *Well if your lungs are gonna be damaged then I don't care if mine are too*. As we were reversing out of our spot in the car park, so many thoughts were spinning around my head and the tears were close. We were both exhausted in every way possible. All of a sudden there was a loud 'crump' from behind and my thoughts were jolted out the window. We'd hit another car! I rolled my eyes and swore through clenched teeth. *Bloody hell, that's all we bloody need.*

So, a devastating diagnosis and car crash later, I was bathing our brave little boy (and trying not to imagine bacteria attacking your tiny lungs), when daddy flumped onto the settee, beer in hand, and sighed, 'At least it was nothing to do with our age.'

I looked at him with a twisted smile. We both started laughing; what else could we do? It was such a surreal situation. While everyone had been so caught up worrying about the much-ballyhooed 'aged parent' risks (chromosomal abnormalities, premature babies, physical disabilities, blah-blah-blah), no-one had been watching out for cystic fibrosis!

Daddy wasn't long in adopting the attitude that there's a lot of worse things out there that you could have; I think that was due to his time working within the care industry, during which he'd seen a lot of severely disabled people living with all sorts of things. 'It's not as though he's in a wheelchair, unable to move,' he reasoned. It did balance my fragile, ragged emotions a bit, but it would be a little while before I'd get to the same point as him.

Grieving

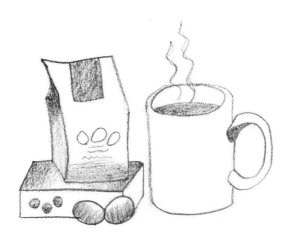

The shock was absolute. I often found myself sitting staring at you, our beautiful little bundle, lying peacefully sleeping in your Moses basket, and wondered how it could be possible. I tried to imagine what was going on inside your tiny body, but just couldn't put the two things together – you and *that*. *How dare it invade your body!* I cried and cried.

One dark evening, shortly after diagnosis, I was settling you in your bed in the nursery when daddy came into the room and pulled me towards him in a silent hug. Tears welled in my eyes. 'What was that for?' I whispered.

'Cos it's so sad. He's your little son.'

The tears were no longer in my eyes and I sobbed and sobbed. So many appointments and medicines. It was extremely overwhelming.

The doctor we saw at the hospital phoned days after our initial visit; I was also getting texts from the nurse but I didn't want to reply to them or speak with any of them, so daddy had to deal with all that. He seemed a lot more emotionally able to cope with it all than I could, on the surface at any rate. It felt like the doctor was checking on us and ascertaining our state of mind and how we were processing everything. We'd briefly scanned the information leaflets they'd given us then put them in a drawer. Out of sight. Seeing the cold, stark words in print was just a reminder we couldn't cope with yet.

A few days after your diagnosis, the nurse came to the house with a bag of medication. The bag was marked with your name which made me very sad. *So, it's final then. Official.* I felt like you were some horrid piece of NHS property now. That sticker on the bag with your name made me feel annoyed, as if they thought they owned you or something; seems daft now but that's how I felt at the time. I wanted the nurse out of our house and to never come back. However, she was here and she would be back – we just had to get used to this new turn of events. She went over the medication you'd be taking on a daily basis – flucloxacillin antibiotic, abidec multivitamins and vitamin E. I could make my peace with the vitamins; many babies need extra vitamins and, hell, even we took vitamin pills, but the antibiotics bothered me a lot. I really didn't want to put that stuff into you. I saw it as poison. This was going to be a struggle for me, and I dreaded to think how I was supposed to even get you to take it. It seemed quite a lot for a baby, and I supposed it would likely taste vile. It was all a bit daunting and I felt profoundly sad that you needed all this.

Daddy's folks came round a couple of days after diagnosis to generously lend us one of their cars so that you and I could use our own car to get out and about when daddy was at work.   (This mainly meant visiting my mum. Spending time back out at her house helped me feel slightly more sane and able to cope with it all.   I could switch off a little and subconsciously put myself back in time to when I lived there; it helped, it really did.   Until I remembered again. *I don't live here and I have a baby with cystic fibrosis.   Shit, I need to deal with this.*)   During their visit, they mentioned a friend of theirs who have a grand-daughter with cystic fibrosis.   She was now nine years old and "doing really well." They had a lot of positive things to say about the condition, such as all the scientific advances being made these days and how, with the correct treatment, people are living much longer now.   They reinforced what the team at the hospital had said (*the more it's said, the more it'll sink in, right?   I hope so*).   We (well, when I say 'we' it was probably more me than daddy) did some Google-ing ourselves, which can be a bit addictive and not always very productive. We had been advised by the team to stick to the Cystic Fibrosis Trust website as it's the go-to organisation with the most reliable, up-to-date and trustworthy information out there, for the UK.   Even with all this hopeful conversation, I felt blue and dazed.

'But *we* passed it on to him…' I couldn't get that out of my head. It was *our* fault!

'You didn't know.' they replied softly.

Their comforting words and tone brought tears to my eyes. I looked away as my lips started to tremble. Tears were never far from my eyes in those early days.

Like many newborns, you were sometimes difficult to settle back to sleep after a night feed. On some nights, it could take one or two hours of constant crying before you finally went back to sleep, but then you'd want fed again a couple of hours later. I would be completely shattered on those nights; I'd often drift off myself, only to wake with a jolt some time later to find you asleep on top of me – those early days and nights can be a real shock for first time parents! One dreadful night when you wouldn't go back to sleep after a feed, mere days after your diagnosis, you were lying in my arms crying your head off. I felt so exhausted and yes, probably a bit depressed. Suddenly I found myself staring down at your tiny little body and all I could think was, *You are going to die. You have things wrong inside your body and you are going to die!* I was still in such confused shock. My chest tightened, a lump rose in my throat and I cried until I fell asleep, utterly worn out.

I spent many late evenings looking out the window onto the deserted street, waiting on daddy to return from work; tears running down my cheeks in silence, my heart breaking. I kept thinking about cystic fibrosis and how on earth had we been carriers and how bad was our luck that we both passed the faulty gene on? I cried a lot in those quiet moments; so sad and angry at God, the universe, whoever, whatever. I didn't know who or what I believed in anymore to be honest. I was still in shock and couldn't accept this had happened. You had had more chance of *not* getting it (the statistics: 50% chance of being a carrier only, 25% of not even being a carrier and 25% of having cystic fibrosis. One in four chance basically). I just didn't want you to have a complicated life or to die young. I tried to remember anything positive we'd been told, to give me hope and strength to get through the next day. In my hazy brain, one thing I could remember the nurse saying was, 'His lungs are perfect just now, just like any other baby's. The aim is to keep them that way for as long as possible; to prevent infection, which is why he is getting the antibiotics, and to help him remove the sticky mucus, which is where the physiotherapy comes in.' I've gone through the grieving process before and know all the stages and how awful it can be, so it's not lost on me that I was grieving at that point – grieving the loss of a perfectly healthy baby who would lead a perfectly healthy, normal life. At least that's how I saw it back then; now I know you *are* perfect and normal and that you will live a *fantastic* life.

Your granny (my mum) started to come round a lot after your diagnosis, when daddy was working. I guess she didn't like the thought of us being alone. She stayed all evening; we had supper together, granny on the settee and me on my birth ball with you strapped into the baby sling, sound asleep. We'd watch episodes of *Everybody Loves Raymond* which did cheer me up and remove me from my current reality. She brought me tons of chocolate at my request (*Well, if I can't smoke......*) but did worry about how much crap I was eating. At one point, she advised I be careful cos I'm breastfeeding and basically nourishing you as well. I took more stock after that, and my diet improved from chocolate, cups of tea, water, breakfast and the odd decent meal, to something much more balanced. I do this when I'm grieving: I think I'm ok with it all then it hits me that actually, no, I'm not ok. Bad news never seems to get any easier to bear.

It was a sign of the depression stage of grief, but I knew it was a phase. I knew I'd pull myself together and step up to this new challenge. It would just take time to get our heads round it. Granny and I talked a lot during those visits, going over and over everything everyone had said and anything we'd read online. She comforted me with logical facts, such as, 'Lots of people depend on medication to keep them healthy, and even alive.' A little bit of perspective goes a long way.

I was still unable to get out of the house much cos of my leg pain, and at times it was so frustrating – it felt as though I was doing everything with one arm (cos the other was holding a crutch) and one leg. The sling did help, as I was hands-free at last (bliss!), but still everything was extremely slow-moving and irritating.

'I feel like I'm grieving,' I told daddy one afternoon.
He nodded in agreement.

'But grieving what?'
'Well,' he replied, 'you have to try and figure out what's making you feel like that.'

After a short pause, I replied, 'Grieving the loss of our healthy child.'

That's how it felt at the beginning; but I also knew that you were our beautiful son, and you would be healthy. I just had to work through the tears and sadness and figure out how to cope and live this new way.

Perhaps you will be my inspiration, I thought. *Perhaps you will show me the silver lining to this dark cloud over us. Perhaps **you** will be the silver lining.*

If we thought it was bad having the midwives and health visitors always coming round in those first days after we brought you home, things were about to get a lot worse.

Blood, Sweat and Tears

X-Ray Reception

We had been advised to keep an eye on your poop: there were signs to look out for that might indicate you weren't absorbing your food well enough. Nutrition is very important in cystic fibrosis, and gaining weight was a good sign. We were informed that – historically – people with cystic fibrosis would struggle to put on weight and would often *look* ill; however the discovery and addition of the digestive enzymes to the diet was something of a breakthrough in cystic fibrosis treatment. Not everyone needs them though, only those who are 'pancreatic insufficient'. Due to your genetic variation, they anticipated that you would be. At our initial appointment, they had taken a sample of your poop to confirm whether or not you were pancreatic insufficient (basically, whether or not you had enough digestive juices getting through the sticky mucus of your pancreas), but held off on the enzymes for now. I pinned my hopes quite a bit on your pancreas working as that would mean you wouldn't need those 'hundreds and thousands' added to every feed. It would be great if that was ok and stayed ok, if it was 'just' your lungs. I didn't know if it worked like that though. They were happy enough that you were weight-gaining and your poop didn't show any of the tell-tale signs of poor absorption. These were the warning signs to look out for:

- Green poop
- Strange smell
- Oily

- Greasy
- Wouldn't float if flushed down toilet (hard to tell while in nappies, will be easier to tell as you get older)
- More poop than considered normal

You were to go back to the hospital for another procedure called a 'sweat test': this would confirm the diagnosis (people with cystic fibrosis have a higher level of chloride in their sweat, which, incidentally, also makes their skin taste a bit salty). The nurse said that although it's a routine procedure, they already knew that you had cystic fibrosis. She sometimes came across as smug to me, and I wanted to slap her. But I know now that she was just doing her job and it was my denial that was skewing my perspective. You would also get a scan and chest x-ray. It seemed an awful lot all at once, and too much for a month old baby. It was really quite a dreadful time. Trying to be strong for each other, as well as ourselves, but confused and a bit adrift at the same time. I felt a bit lonely and isolated within my own mind. Very hard to explain, and I hope to never have to go through those feelings again.

One slightly positive bit of news was that you would be on the antibiotics for at least three years, then the aim would be to take you off them and monitor you without. The reason you were given antibiotics was what they call 'prophylactic' – intended to *prevent* infection. As the nurse put it, 'To put a protective blanket around your lungs.' It's not that you had lots of bugs on your lungs: it's to try to keep them away. It did take me a few months for all that to sink in, to be honest. I think I had to be told on several different occasions before I understood.

You would have monthly clinic appointments for a while until your treatment plan had settled into place, then they would be every three months, and finally once a year when you were a bit older. Along with these, the nurse also explained that you'd be getting annual reviews, which included x-rays, scans and blood tests. While I found it difficult to cope with knowing you needed all this observation, granny assured me that you were in safe hands, our beautiful baby boy. The nurse said the aim was for all babies diagnosed at birth now to have a life expectancy of seventy years. Well, no-one can sniff at that kind of lifespan. I felt a bit more comforted when she said things like that. All we could do was hope for the future, but try not to think too far ahead as we had enough to be getting on with in the present. Rest our hopes for the future in the hands of the clever scientists for now.

Giving the first dose of antibiotics was, as dreaded, difficult to do to you (*to* you, not *for* you, as I see it now. It was early days). I had to wake you up for it. It seemed so much to give at one time and you did protest and didn't swallow it all, which was understandable as you

47

were just used to breast milk. It made me sick to my stomach that you were having to be force fed this pink, bitter stuff when a baby should only have to drink warm, sweet milk. It about broke my heart thinking about it. Yes, it was a big stress for us all, such a hard thing to do to a tiny baby.

It wasn't the first time I'd felt that way, though: syringes were nothing new to me as I'd done some intensive nursing with several pets in the past, which was just as traumatic and stressful and I hated being reminded of those dreadful days. However, I think that experience helped me realise that I could do this and we could get through this. Subconsciously, I think, I started referring to your condition as CF instead of cystic fibrosis – it felt much less scary and fatalistic; it almost sounded benign that way.

One morning I was breastfeeding you when I got another call from the nurse (I hated seeing her name come up on my phone. I wished she would call daddy but I was the main caregiver so I had to get used to this sooner or later). The cough swab taken at the hospital had come back showing you'd grown a bacterium called staphylococcus aureus on your lungs. I was told it wasn't a serious infection, but they wanted to catch and treat it. *Bloody hell, how can you have something already?!* I had to give you a double dose of flucloxacillin for two weeks – four times a day for two weeks! *How in the hell will we do that?* I felt sick and wobbly, feeling slightly unable to cope. Depressing. *Why on earth is this happening, and why should a baby so young have to put up with this? What poisons am I having to give my precious boy?* (In time, I would start to think of the antibiotics as our friend, rather than our enemy). I wanted the nurse to stop phoning and texting, to leave us alone. Oh, I really hated having her in my life. While I fell apart, she remained completely professional.

'At least we've caught it early and can treat it.'

Daddy agreed.
I was struggling, I'm afraid.
My poor boy.
Not fair.

I felt angry at the nurse – at all of them – for being right about you having this. I so desperately wanted them to be wrong, that this was a weird, horrid dream.

Of course, throughout all of this trauma, I still had hellish leg pain and that disability to contend with. The physiotherapy exercises weren't helping, so I'd decided to visit an independent osteopath. Before we left for my first appointment, I'd had a private cry in the house: you wouldn't settle, I'd not had much time to get ready and I was so upset about having to give you the antibiotics. Daddy gave me a hug. I felt drained. I was also texting my mum for support and strength. Everyone in our lives was great – full of love, kindness and positivity.

Our heads were still buzzing with everything when daddy drove us there; you still such a tiny baby in the car seat, dwarfed by your sleep suit. While in consultation with the very compassionate lady, we decided that explaining the bigger picture of our circumstances was relevant to my overall health and state of mind, so we revealed your diagnosis. Yes, I did cry a little when we had that conversation with her; I always start crying when things are emotional and someone speaks in soothing, understanding tones. (As you'll realise when you're older, mummy is a bit of an emotional doily). However, whilst she said we sounded sad, we also sounded rational and we *were* coping. Even if it did not feel like it.

The appointment went well, and I finally started to feel like someone was taking proper interest in my leg and I could get to the bottom of it. I'd started to worry that I'd always be like this, but that would be impossible for me; I have far too much to do to be hobbling about on one leg. Just give me the hip op if that's what it takes. The osteopath reassured me that I wasn't a lost cause; she wasn't sure what had happened yet, but she was certain she could figure it out or refer me to someone who could. As positive as that was, for me physically anyway, I think I must have used up all my remaining energy on acting as normal and sociable as possible in that appointment, cos when I got back to the car and daddy drove out of there, all I could think about was you needing double antibiotics already. Was this how it was going to be, so soon? There you were, asleep in your car seat, totally unaware that you had bacteria bugs attacking your tiny little lungs; the perfect little lungs that daddy and mummy had made together. It was more than I could bear, and I cried silently behind sunglasses all the way home. I never told daddy about that until a year later. He had had no idea.

We got all sorts of missed calls and texts in the early days as things were trying to settle into a routine (not a routine we wanted, but there it was anyway). I would get missed calls from our GP, asking about the antibiotic strength for your prescription. Oh, how I longed for every call and text to be someone telling me they'd made a mistake and you didn't have CF.

We had the date for the sweat test, x-ray and scan. Of course, I was hoping against all the odds that the sweat test would come back negative, but I guess I knew that it wouldn't. You were a very good boy for the tests, much better than mummy who hated all those people poking and prodding you. The sweat test didn't hurt; it was just a contraption similar to a blood pressure band around your arm that apparently induced sweat, with tubes attached that collected the sweat as it ran through them. Obviously you didn't enjoy it and were a bit wriggly, but all-in-all you handled it well. Again, much better than mummy. At one point after they were done, the CF nurse wanted to hold you while I fumbled about for your snowsuit; I almost screamed 'Let go of my baby! Get your hands off him!!' Close to tears of confusion, emotional exhaustion and - yes - probably anger, I felt so out of my comfort zone in there. I hated them all knowing about your condition and that you were just another statistic or something. *He's our beautiful baby boy and he doesn't belong in here! He should be at home without needles and tubes and x-rays! This is all wrong!* The doctor who did the ultrasound said that everything looked normal, which perked us up a bit, but when the CF doctor and nurse came in and started talking digestive enzymes and you probably needing them, I felt deflated again. I hated seeing those two; I wanted to slap their faces. I was ready to walk out of the room if that doctor didn't shut up; I could've thrown my water cup at him. *Wish he'd shut up about CF stuff! I hate coming into this place!*

We were informed that people with CF are advised to avoid close contact with one another. This is due to the risks of cross-infection occurring between them, potentially causing serious harm to their health. If in the future you want to talk to someone with CF, you can do it remotely via online chats, email, Skype, phone calls, texts, etc. We were also informed that, as part of the team's on-going care plan, if we moved to another area they would notify the CF unit nearest to us for a smooth transition. All units are aware of how many children with CF reside in their area, and where they live. This is especially helpful for nursery and school, to keep the risks of cross-infection to a minimum. Apparently, if there is more than one child with CF in a school, they are advised to use separate classrooms. Although I see it all clearer now, and understand the importance of such attention to detail, at that time it just felt like you were being treated like a leper or something: *Watch out, people, he's coming! Run!* Or if we go swimming, are we to yell out, 'Anyone here with CF? No? Good, we're safe.' Geez, depressing.

I remember one evening after the scans and sweat test, I was in the shower trying to visualise daddy coming in and telling me the doctor had phoned to say it had all been a mistake; they'd checked your results, and you didn't have cystic fibrosis after all. Of course, that didn't happen. These were the desperate thoughts coming and going from my mind in those early days post diagnosis. The denial stage of grief.

Even with all this going on, I managed to get some nice relaxing baths while daddy dozed with you downstairs. If we were lucky, you would sleep in your Moses basket long enough for me to get a soak in the tub or grab three or four hours' sleep. My leg pain had to take a back seat priority-wise now; just another challenge to work through. What doesn't kill you, as they say! I started to have some quite insightful perspectives early on, such as both you and us using this diagnosis to our advantage: when you're aware of your mortality and that you may have a shorter lifespan/sell-by-date, you can make the most of life and do all the things you fancy. Most people probably take life for granted and don't make the most of their time here; they don't appreciate their mortality until it's too late. Enjoy it while you can…?

I worried about little things, such as whether or not it was ok to give this flucloxacillin with a breastfeed, as the bottle said to give on an empty stomach. But you try telling that to a baby when they wake up wanting fed! 'Sorry, sweetie, but you'll have to wait an hour after your meds before I can feed you.' Yea, right. These were just some of the practicalities and challenges that we had to navigate. Trial and error, I suppose. I did check with the nurse and she assured us it was fine to give it near a feed with a baby as this was often the only practicable way to do it; imagine how much more complicated it got when you had picked up some bug in your lungs and needed it four times a day!

You were starting to interact with us more, seeing more and smiling a bit when we made silly voices. I still had to work at accepting you had this condition; it was hard but I had to move on. I was starting to feel the fight in me. *I will try to let go of my preconceived image of how I saw your early life. I will try to make everything right for you, baby.*

I was still hoping that your digestive system would be ok, but the doctor had said you have the 'classic' gene so you probably *will* need the enzymes. I still had my fingers crossed for a bit of luck, though; hell, we were due it.

Every now and then, even at this early stage, I would get glimpses of feeling a bit better – almost (dare I say it?) 'normal'. I enjoyed some hysterical laughing with granny as she kept miserably failing to take some photos of you and me with my phone camera. A bit silly, but really this was my first proper laugh in days since, well…..you know. Daddy gave you your antibiotics that evening, while you slept, which was quite successful. While I had moments of feeling more able to cope, I knew that it could all change in an instant so I was always a little bit on edge with my emotions at that point. I didn't trust them yet.

I felt very scared to read anything about CF online, and was very cautious when I did feel brave enough to do so. I'd read about older sufferers and how they took their meds, and it seemed more manageable than what we were doing at the moment. I felt sure it would get easier; they seemed to have almost normal lives. What's normal anyway? Of course, in between moments of clarity and light, there were still the awful moments of feeling overwhelmed with your diagnosis and the amount of meds you needed.

My mum thought that the medical staff were just being extra cautious as 'they won't want to lose him.' And at the start it'll feel like they're all up in our faces (yes!) but it will get easier – they'll probably have less interaction as we get more used to it all and with what we're doing. Oh, I really did hope so. I remembered sitting listening to them that first evening in the hospital, thinking, *Am I really here? Is this happening? Is he talking to us*? With each day, I had no idea how I'd feel until it happened. And I didn't know when that would get easier.

I can smell those awful antibiotics. I hate the bloody stuff. You take it, but often cry. It breaks me.

The day after the sweat test, I had a missed call from the nurse. I had no intention of speaking with her, so daddy called her back.

56

Sweat test confirms diagnosis. I guess I had been expecting – hoping for – a miracle somehow. *The next nightmare will be the enzymes. God, when will he have time to do anything else other than take bloody medication. It's all wrong.* Nothing felt like it should have. How I wished my only problems were a crying baby and a dodgy leg, like it had been only a week earlier!

I felt so angry.
And confused.
How the hell did this happen?
Is this a nightmare?
When can I wake up?
What's next?
Your daddy dying?
Your granny dying?
The dog?
One of the cats?
Bloody hell.

I felt like someone had taken my life, shaken it, and thrown the pieces into the wind. Good luck finding them again.

Some days I was sure that your poop smelled, which was a bad sign. *Oh God, can't his digestive system just be ok? Can't his pancreas just be producing enzymes – please!!* That horrible doctor said you'd probably need enzymes; we'd passed on the 'classic gene' and most people with that need them. I wondered if they relished a new diagnosis. Like a new statistic. I hated them. *Stop bothering me! I don't want to hear any more about it!* I felt so blue again.

I'm sorry, baby.

I'm sorry that we have to give you that putrid stuff.

I'm sorry we gave you CF.

Masks, Meds and Syringes

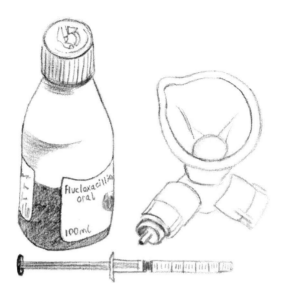

I got to be so concerned with your weight; desperate for you to put on weight and for your poop to be ok, cos if you didn't or if it wasn't, they'd want you on those enzymes. However, I tried not to put too much emphasis or expectation on your weight gains. Even though it felt like good news to me, I was too scared to trust anything in those early days, as we'd had so much bad news in such a short space of time, so much to take in and come to terms with; I felt I couldn't cope with much more on top of all this. We didn't have scales, but your granny did, so I would weigh you at her house in between the health visitor's weight checks. This gave me a lot of confidence and reassurance that you *were* putting on weight. Granny could tell that you were growing, but it was harder for me to see subtle changes like that, I suppose cos I was with you all the time. I went with how quickly you grew out of your clothes, while trying not to let the weigh-ins become an obsession. I so desperately didn't want you on the digestive enzymes – not yet anyway. *If he will need them, please just don't let it be yet. It's too much.*

Daddy got a phone call from the doctor at the hospital (thank God he didn't call me), to basically say that the blood and sweat tests didn't reveal anything different.

'So, no new horrors then?' sighed daddy.

To me, it just meant that you didn't *not* have it. They weren't wrong. I guess I just hoped that they were. 'It'll come,' daddy assured me.

The nurse had put us in touch with a charity called The Butterfly Trust, who supported families dealing with CF. They helped with all sorts of things – such as benefits, counselling, grants, support, etc. I was immediately impressed and deeply grateful that such a charity existed for one specific health condition. Following my initial email to them, I was surprised when a support worker offered to come to our house to chat things over and fill out some forms. That was a huge load off us, not just the help with benefit applications (which would absolutely have been too much to cope with), but also that we weren't going to have to leave the comfort of home at this emotionally frayed time, not to mention the physical difficulties of travelling to their office with my leg in the state it was. The support worker sounded nice; they were there to support us in any way. I felt a little weight was lifted from my heavy shoulders.

You were still on double dose antibiotics at this point, and sometimes you cried even when I gave you the vitamins. Yes, they were quite a small dose compared to the antibiotics, but they still seemed far too much to put into a tiny baby's mouth. Because you were so young, you would often be asleep when antibiotic time came round again, so I would slide the tip of the syringe into the side of your little mouth and gently push the plunger in as you slept. You didn't wake up, making it surprisingly easy to do. It made me feel a *bit* better about it. The Butterfly Trust support worker reminded me that no matter how hard it was to do to you, it was *preventative*. I was glad of the reminder, as it seemed more comforting to know that it was to protect you from damage, rather than actually treating damage that was already there. Remember the nurse's words: 'His lungs are perfect just now, just like any other baby's'.

There were all sorts of 'teething' problems at this early stage; one day I might find it relatively simple to administer your meds with little to no protest from you, and the next day you might take your meds screaming then vomit them up moments later. A learning curve, that's for sure. As frustrating as it was, I felt we had to adapt quite quickly and get on with it, cos it needed to be done. No point lingering on the negative too long as that wouldn't change one damn thing. That said, I slid (or settled) into a kind of numb-like state; administer your meds whilst ignoring your condition as best I could. That really helped me start to see you as our healthy little boy again. Some (most welcome) perspective would often creep in as well, from myself or from others, such as *plenty people have to take medication to stay alive.*

When you were one month old, we enjoyed making hand and foot prints with you, and taking photos to mark the occasion. Normal new parent activities; nothing to do with any genetic conditions or medication. *Things aren't so bad*, I told myself. *No matter what's going on inside you, we might have the sweetest, most perfect and loving child here; the most sweet, perfect, loving, loyal, caring, compassionate human. And wouldn't that be much more important than physically perfect?* Who is physically perfect anyway?

Your auntie thinks they'll find a cure soon. I wasn't very clued up yet on all the current research and breakthroughs being made, although the nurse had waxed lyrical about that on her visit. And even though I didn't quite understand, I sensed the extremely positive vibe from her, and that did help ease some of my pain. I still didn't want to know too much, in terror of more bad news, but anything hopeful was welcome news (even though the gist was enough information for me at that point).

Always watching your nappies, I'd feel myself getting a bit panicky when I thought your poop was especially smelly or a bit green-looking. *Damn it!* I'd mutter, while Google-imaging what green poop might mean and what normal, healthy poop should look like. Yes, that page was open on my laptop quite a lot!

Family were brilliant at keeping our spirits up in those early days; I really don't know how we would've coped without such a positive support network. They certainly kept me buoyed up on my worst days.

'There will be lots of progress with research by the time he's a teenager,' one sister said. She went on to say that even she'd been taking enzymes at one point, as she'd felt like food was just sitting in her stomach and not being digested properly.

'Things won't be as bad as you imagine,' she continued. And you know what, just months on as it turned out, they really weren't.

One of the few friends we opened up to about your condition was really supportive and non-dramatic about it. She told me how most days she needed to use her inhaler for asthma, and that made me feel better. It made me feel like we were less isolated and disabled than I'd thought. While some people feel offended if their condition is described as 'not so bad' or 'could be worse', I felt much better cos it indicated to me that they don't think it's so bad. And that, in turn, comforted me. I could relax cos *it's not so bad; there are definitely worse things out there*. I can't imagine having any other attitude about it; I don't want to feel like it's something awful. It is what it is and there's not much you can do about that. Why make it worse by seeing only the negatives?

We were a bit surprised about you having to start physio and (potentially) enzymes so soon if your lungs were healthy just now, but realised that it's preventative – to protect you and *keep* you that way as long as possible. If we focus on that, then we can just about cope with it all. I think the fact that CF is quite a hidden condition really helps with the coping; at that age anyway, there were no outward indications that anything was wrong with you, so no-one need know. Certainly, in those early months, it greatly helped me 'forget'; *do what I need to do, but don't dwell on it.* Would I have been able to do that, or get to that stage of acceptance so quickly, if you had had physical signs of a health condition? I don't know. Perhaps. But I think that would have made it an even more difficult journey to navigate. Yes, we love our children as they are, but that doesn't mean it's easy to accept, or easy to cope, when things aren't as we'd expected them to be. But love will conquer all, I do believe that. It just sometimes takes a bit of time. And I'm not going to pretend it's any other way. I can only speak for us, and it did take time to accept it or 'get over' it and move on with normal parenthood. Of course we love you unconditionally, we always have (and always will), but we did have to work through our grief. Funnily enough, as it turns out, things are much easier to deal with than I'd ever thought possible back then. In fact, some days I wonder what all the fuss was about!

When you were a month old, the nurse came out to our house again, this time with the physiotherapist. Daddy was at work, so I was going to be on my own with them. *God, I hope they don't stay long!* I still found home visits extremely intrusive, disruptive and stressful. I was still resisting the fact that these people were in our lives, and still did not like them. The meeting was ok, though; I might even have ever so slightly warmed to them. The need for physio was explained as 'airway clearance' – we all have mucus in our lungs but, with CF, the mucus is thicker and stickier and that's where bugs thrive. You need physio to help remove this mucus on a daily basis. I was shown your physio mask, known as a PEP (Positive Expiratory Pressure) mask. It was in three parts that we put together: the mask, a pressure resistor and a three part valve. The resistor keeps the airways open and makes you exhale with a bit more effort than normal breathing, and this pressure forces the air under any pockets of mucus stuck in the lungs, enabling it to be removed from the lungs and either swallowed or spat out. PEP therapy allows more air to reach the smaller airways in the lungs. The physiotherapist tried it out with you, while explaining how it worked. All-in-all you did two minutes PEP and did really well. Of course it highly bothered me to see my baby with a rubber mask over his nose and mouth, but the more numb I tried to remain, the more I could cope with each new step. You'd eaten before they came, so I think you were really relaxed. It gave me a false sense of security, I have to admit; things were *not* going to be that effortless moving forward. She explained that we should aim for five minutes a day. Start with one minute of the mask, rest a minute or two, one minute of the mask, rest, and so on, building up to a total of five one-minute sessions of breathing into the mask.

Before they left, the nurse gave me some encouraging news: scientists are currently working on drugs that act on a cellular level for the F508del variation that you have; 'they have it', she nodded, 'they just need to perfect it.' I felt a lot more upbeat about it all than I had yet. I prayed that it continued.

So, it's all about masks, medication and syringes now. Around this time, I lost the fight with The Constantly Crying Baby and succumbed to The Dummy. At first you weren't keen, which was a big disappointment. I'd never intended to use dummies, but I guess there comes a point when you literally can't take the screaming one minute longer. I had no idea how exhausting all that noise would be. I don't think the pressures of CF had anything to do with our decision to use a dummy (or soother as they seem to be called now). I just didn't have the headspace for any more of that piercing crying and didn't know what else to do about it; we'd tried everything else. When you took the dummy and happily sucked on it, the resulting peace was bliss! Rightly or wrongly, there it was, and I could only hope that you'd be ok without it now. This was all new to me.

PEP at this point was a bit hit and miss, but still relatively quiet (though that was about to change). Sometimes I put it over your face as you slept; I figured it didn't really matter right now if you were awake or not, as long as you were getting your chest physio. I knew it couldn't always be done that way, but we were all still very new to it and anything I could do to ease the stress for us, I grabbed with both hands. I kind of dreaded it to be honest, waiting for you to start crying when the mask went on, which started to happen very quickly and the sound broke my heart.

I made sure we had a few baths together while you were still young enough to enjoy the skin-to-skin contact and closeness. It was a fantastic feeling to breastfeed you in the water then let you fall asleep in my arms, against my skin. You seemed to enjoy being held in the water, and didn't seem afraid, which made me feel proud cos I wanted you to grow up to be a water baby. Throughout all of this CF nightmare, I will never forget the loving, beautiful, tender moments of motherhood;

moments that reminded me that we had the most amazing gift of all in our precious child. Moments that united me with all other parents, no matter what they may or may not be going through in their journey.

Along with the constant worry of how much you were eating - *you need to eat to keep putting on weight, baby!* – the administration of antibiotics started to get more difficult as you resisted with almost each syringe. There were little upsets along the way with meds, such as the pharmacy being out of the usual one (with added sugar for a more palatable taste) and us having to take an alternative (sugar free and very bitter). Unexpected switches like this were just an added stress, to be honest, and you were the least impressed of all. After several texts to the nurse, we did manage to get back to the added sugar antibiotic, which was easier for you to swallow. *You're my baby and I've got your back.* In addition to that, it did take our pharmacy and GP practice a bit of time to understand all the instructions coming from the hospital, especially as it regarded antibiotics (which are not usually prescribed on a weekly basis, so required a bit of explanation). We were extremely glad when things settled into a weekly routine of the GP sending the prescriptions to the chemist for us, making one less thing to worry about. We would regularly get annoyed about these things in those days though, not understanding why we couldn't just have what we needed and why life couldn't be a bit simpler and give us a damn break.

Nowadays, of course, you're a lot bigger and take to these changes much easier when they happen, which in turn makes it much easier on us. But, back then, it made me dread meds time and having to put all that horrid stuff into your mouth as you screamed, with actual tears rolling down your face. It made me feel like a bad mother, the way you looked at me with pleading eyes; you might as well have been screaming, *'No, mummy, no!'*

As if dealing with a heart breaking diagnosis wasn't hard enough, putting my baby through all this pain and stress was like shit icing on a fetid cake.

You were ok once the meds were in; it was just traumatic for us both to administer. I felt like it would be much easier to give via a spoon, at least you'd see it coming then. (As it turned out though, we pretty much stuck with the syringes for your regular antibiotics; it *did* get easier). No matter how careful I was to place the syringe into the side of your mouth and push the plunger very slowly aiming towards your cheek, you still momentarily choked a little sometimes. I guess it just wasn't something you were anticipating. I knew it would probably get easier as you got older, when I could tell you it was coming, or perhaps you'd just get used to it on your own.

Either way, that was in the future but at that time it was very stressful and it pained me to have to do that to you. I knew, deep down (I still struggled with it), that it was for your own good, but how could I tell a baby that? Again, it reminded me of when I gave meds to several pets; you can't tell them or a baby, 'Here comes your meds, get ready!' I tried to soothe you with my voice as best I could. Luckily, you did settle afterwards, as though nothing had happened. The timing of meds also remained an issue; I was aware it was best to give it on an empty stomach, but that was near impossible with a baby. Besides, it often comforted you to have a feed afterwards and I felt the benefit of that was more important. We had been assured it was fine at your age to give it with food, and that was good enough for us. We didn't have a whole hell of a lot of choice anyway, to be honest.

PEP physio gradually increased to four minutes with the mask, although I did sometimes still do it after you'd fallen asleep. Baby steps, as they say. Better than not doing it at all. We'd get there. Slowly but surely, we managed to take it to my birth ball (I was glad to have bought one during pregnancy as the physiotherapist was highly in favour of them for chest physio), bouncing gently while watching some baby music on the laptop for distraction. Some days you barely cried at all, and along with the days where you took your meds easier, I felt a little bit more, *hey, this isn't so bad.*

I was still clinging to the hope that if your poop was normal and you were gaining weight, you wouldn't need the digestive enzymes. The same day that you finished your double dose of antibiotics – *thank goodness and please let the bug be gone and you don't get another one for ages* – we had a home visit from the dietician. There were no big surprises at this initial visit. She had a look at your nappy and thought it looked normal enough but the result of your poop sample from the hospital would tell if your pancreatic enzymes were getting through or not. Oh, I did hope so! I was to start a breastfeeding chart that she had drawn up, to ascertain how often you were feeding and for how long. We had to watch out for you eating more than usual because that could indicate that your body wasn't absorbing sufficient nutrients: guzzling more and more to try and fill yourself. And there was me worrying about you *not eating enough food*. I kept on with my pee and poop 'diary' as well as now keeping track of your feeds. As the dietician was leaving the house, I mentioned the dreaded digestive enzymes, asking if there was a chance you may not need them. 'Fingers crossed,' she said with a smile that gave me hope, cos it wasn't a no.

PEP physio continued to grow into a bit of a trial. Most times you would cry at some point during it, often falling asleep after you were cried out, letting me finish as you slept. I was still of the mind that this way was less stress for both of us and I didn't see the harm in it at this stage. The mask momentarily left a horrible red mark around your little baby face afterwards, which pulled at my heart and made me feel so sad for you. *My beautiful little boy, you shouldn't have to go through all of this!* And what a beautiful smiley boy you were growing into. You loved me singing rhymes to you, as well as songs such as 'Yes Sir, I can Boogie'. There's no accounting for taste eh?

Daddy had introduced me to the wonders of Milton sterilising tablets, which I used for your syringes and your PEP equipment after thoroughly washing them in warm soapy water. That way, syringes could be used more than once and the PEP was as sterile as I could possibly make it. After every use, they were cleaned in this way; of course I didn't know if this was going a bit overboard, but better to be safe than sorry I reckoned. Drying it was a bit of a learning curve; kitchen roll and towels left tiny dust particles on the mask, which would be inhaled, so blow drying or air drying were the best options.

As you were so young, giving you your meds often woke you from a sleep, poor soul. Oh, how sad it made me to put those syringes into your gummy, toothless mouth. One day I had the brainwave of trying to give you the morning antibiotic at the same time as the abidec and vitamin E, in the hope that this might make the antibiotic more palatable for you (as you already tolerated the vitamins). However, instead of it making you not mind all three, it made you dislike all three. Ugh – worth a try. Never mind, once you'd been fed, changed and were all dummied-up again, you were happy. Onwards and upwards.

Every now and then I'd have a missed call from the nurse at the hospital. *Not calling her back, don't want to speak with her – it's never good news. She'll just have to contact daddy and he can tell me.* More often than not, at this stage of getting settled into our routine, it was just something along the lines of the hospital communicating with our GP to arrange your repeat prescription. But I still felt on a knife edge, dreading more bad news each time my phone beeped or rang. We did have the nurse coming back to do a repeat cough swab though. *God, please let it be clear this time. I really don't want to put you through four antibiotic doses again.*

One day, we won't have to hide from the CF anymore.
Cos it won't matter anymore.
It will be irrelevant.
These days now, they are the hardest.
For you and us.
It will only get better and easier from here.

Little Things

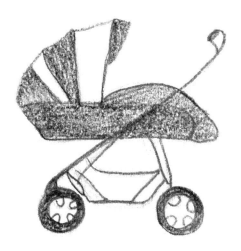

The health visitor came round on a semi-regular basis to do weight and developmental checks. You were still putting on weight, which made me happy for the rest of that day.

'He's above the game,' she smiled, 'good eye contact, smiling, aware of surroundings. All credit to you and your husband, this is really good. It's an exciting time you're coming into.' I could see that as you were starting to do more and interact more, becoming more and more smiley and chatty, our happy sweet little fellow.

The nurse came to do your repeat cough swab and our dog acted a little strange with her. 'I'm going to be here often,' she said patting doggie's head, 'we'll be friends.'

Now, that would have really irritated me a few weeks ago, the thought of her being at our house often enough to be friends with the dog, but it didn't bother me much. I felt better about things. A bit anyway. She reminded me that you would be on the antibiotics until you were three years old then they'd aim to take you off them and only give if needed; if you had an infection. That made my heart sing, every time I heard it or thought about it. Good news. After she'd left, I took you and the dog and headed off to granny's with a smile on my face and a smile in my heart.

PEP was steadily getting more and more stressful as we worked up to the recommended five minutes, you were actually screaming now. At its worst, you would look up at me with a red face and pleading eyes and I swear that it actually sounded like you were sobbing, 'Mummy!' Absolutely horrid, it broke my heart and I almost cried myself. *It's amazing how long one minute feels when you're just praying for it to be over.* Daddy and I got through a lot of comedies, such as *Steptoe and Son*, *Some Mothers Do 'Ave 'Em* and *Are You Being Served?* You particularly liked the theme tunes, and for a short time they calmed you as I bounced you in time to the beat, mask on face. But, alas, all good things must end. Still, mummy and daddy enjoyed the comedy while it lasted, and I especially welcomed the feeling of escapism they'd offered. I tell you, there were days where I felt like I wouldn't have the energy, enthusiasm, or love to do everything all over again tomorrow, but it was amazing how it just seemed to come from somewhere to help me cope with another day. I presumed that was a normal reaction to the shock of first-time parenthood.

We were still waiting for your poop sample result when I had another missed call from the nurse; seeing her name on my phone really did make my blood run cold. Unfortunately, it was the result of your repeat cough swab – you'd caught another bug. Not a serious one, but one they like to treat and get rid of as you were more vulnerable; when other babies got it, they wouldn't be treated. *How could you have something again so soon? Is this the way it's going to be?* I was stunned into silence and sadness.

'It's just bacteria that are out there,' she comforted me, 'we can't avoid them all. Sometimes you'll go for ages without anything then you'll get one or two close together.' I felt a bit easier about it, trying to keep the perspective I'd been working so hard on achieving over the past weeks. As she informed me it was called klebsiella, I wondered who came up with these names. I had to pick up the prescription for a new antibiotic called augmentin. At just 1ml twice a day, it didn't seem too much and, as it was a different antibiotic, we didn't have to try and fit in doses four times a day - we could give it with the flucloxacillin, morning and night, which was a lighter load on us all. When I collected it, it was completely different in look and texture to the fluclox and it smelled of strawberries. You took it well.

You were starting to sleep for longer stretches between feeds, five and a half hours was the longest yet. Wow, it seemed so blissfully long. And that's coming from someone who has always loved sleeping and was never all that keen to get out of bed in the morning.

So, trust me, if I can do this baby thing, anyone can! We went for our first long walk in the pram around this time, with my leg starting to gain strength and flexibility. I chose one of our dog-walking routes from pre-baby days and felt bathed in a strong feeling of nostalgic peace and happiness as I strolled along, feeling relaxed and proud to be lulling my beautiful son to sleep.

PEP wasn't improving much, regarding how well you tolerated it. Sometimes you cried, sometimes you screamed, sometimes you did neither; sometimes you fell asleep, sometimes you didn't and sometimes you did a mix of all of the above in one session. For a short – but very upsetting – time, you actually screamed and flailed and I found it incredibly difficult to continue, but knew I had to. You even grabbed at my hand to get the mask off your face, but of course you couldn't. That look in your eyes, pleading your mummy to stop! It must have been so uncomfortable for you, poor thing. I could feel your little fingernails digging into my hand. I felt like such a bad mother in those moments; it was absolutely horrid. To say it broke my heart all over again is no exaggeration; I felt my whole body sweating under the pressure and stress. I wished you would just relax and breathe, it was much better on you when you did that. I worried about this experience making a dent in our bonding process: would you trust me less because of this? I tried all sorts to keep you distracted, such as playing peekaboo, bouncing, watching joyful baby rhymes on the laptop, but nothing was foolproof. How I wished there was another way and I could only hope that the physio and meds got easier for you. The good news was that you were always ok afterward, but that didn't stop me hating doing that to you, and hating having to.   Still, I was extremely impressed that you were putting up with it at all, baby, and you never cease to amaze me to this day. Such a strong, brave boy.

Little things like walking to the GP with you in the pram to attend my leg physio, then having a chat with the receptionists, made me feel normal again and that felt really good.   These were positive little steps forward that greatly aided my growing acceptance of our new situation.

All health visitor weight checks were positive too; you were gaining weight and all looked well.
'He's like a porcelain dolly,' gushed one. 'Perfect!'
She didn't need to tell us!

I dreamt that you were suddenly standing and walking. Then you were a bit older, you were blonde. Your feet were all malformed and distorted at weird angles and some of your toes were broken, snapped in half and bleeding. But you didn't seem to notice. I felt that it was all too much. I sat you on the bed and asked if you could feel any pain anywhere – you didn't seem to. I thought, 'His feet were straight when he was born! Why is this happening?'

That was my first dream about you. I was very glad when I woke up.

By two months old you were starting to sleep for six to seven hours a night, which was bliss! And at two months old, we had your first clinic meeting at the hospital. Daddy and I felt nervous about this appointment, not quite sure what to expect. On arrival, we headed to the now-familiar Children's Outpatient Department where a member of staff ushered us to a row of private rooms. On the wall beside each room was a white board with the name of a child. Below the child's name was listed: doctor, nurse, dietician, physiotherapist, psychologist and pharmacist - the team members who we soon came to know well. We spotted your name and went into the room and closed the door behind us, wondering with some anxiety what we were about to face. As is often the case in life, the appointment wasn't half as daunting as we'd anticipated. We were introduced to each team member and went through your treatment plan with each of them, as appropriate. Your scan, x-ray and poop results were discussed.

The main upset (for me anyway; daddy seemed to be of the mind 'if he needs it, he needs it') was that they recommended you start on the digestive enzymes – which were apparently called 'creon'. Despite the fact that you were steadily putting on weight and eating well, which they were happy about, your poop sample had come back indicating you were pancreatic insufficient. They would do another sample to cross-check. My heart sank a little. *All that hoping, eh.* I tried to remain positive and rather numb about it. *I'll do what I have to do and try not to get down about it all. Just one more thing to do and hopefully they won't add anything else to your treatment regime. It should get easier as he gets older*, I kept telling myself.

We did a little bit of PEP physio with mixed success, then the nurse took another cough swab, which I really hoped would be clear for once. Poor lad, you cried and looked at me as if to say 'Help me, mummy!' as she did it. *Oh baby, I'm so sorry!* The heartbreak. We were assured that the cough swabs would get easier as you got bigger. She also informed us that she would only come to the house from now on if we needed her, for the foreseeable future anyway, which felt like music to our ears. It felt like a noose around our necks was being slackened a little; we could get on with our lives and enjoy our baby. Good. They weighed you, measured your length and head circumference.

I dreamt that you were a girl and you said your first word, 'hello' to my mum, sister and her friend. I pretended that it wasn't your first word

85

and that you often said 'hi' to me (you have to say your first word to mummy and daddy!) Everyone was commenting on how beautiful you were.

On the way out of the hospital, daddy nipped into one of the cafes for a takeout coffee. As I waited with you, as far away from the buzz of the public as I could get, a lovely older gentleman approached us. I felt my skin tighten and the adrenalin start to rush through me, *Don't come any closer!* He was ever so nice and I guess he just felt drawn to the little baby in the car seat. 'Can I say hello?' he asked me gently. In my paranoia, I replied quickly, 'Depends what you're in for.' Well, this *was* a hospital full of potential germs, after all. In the end, he got to say hello without getting too close to you. *Mission accomplished, now let's get the hell out of here!* We headed to Dobbies for a cuppa and an escape – to feel a bit normal again. *No, we haven't just been at the hospital.* Denial? Perhaps. But it helped me, particularly, to cope.

Safely back home, a swim-ring that we'd ordered had arrived. We planned to use it in the bath first and, later on, the swimming pool. I mainly hoped that you would enjoy it and that it would make you smile and feel relaxed. Cos God knows you had earned that and deserved that. The clothes all three of us wore to clinic were put in the washing machine and I made sure we all had a good bath/shower too; wash the hospital muck and germs from everything. We continue with this routine, which may not be entirely necessary, but that's just us.

So, we started the dreaded enzymes that evening. We stewed some apples (which turned out to be a little bit lumpy for a baby, so we decided to opt for shop-bought organic purees next time. Yes, I finally figured out where to get hold of apple puree) and estimated the required amount of creon in relation to how long you'd breastfed. It wasn't so hard, you took it well. I did feel a twinge of guilt for feeding you anything other than breast milk at two months old, but what could I do? I had no choice. At least the puree was homemade, and if we got organic from the shop, then it was as healthy and safe as we could get for you.

That night in the big bath you did seem to enjoy your swim-ring. Before bed, I tried to trick you with the PEP mask by only putting the mask without the attachments on your face, to get you used to it. It seemed to work, as you didn't stress so much; the first two minutes you didn't cry, the second two you did cry and by the last minute, you settled.

I was still obsessing over the colour of your poop, looking out for green (which did show up every now and then, freaking me out). I guess I really did think that if your poop looked healthy and you kept putting on weight, then you didn't need the enzymes. If only it were that simple. But the day after starting creon, I texted the nurse saying we'd like to hold off on it until we could get that second poop sample they talked about at clinic, for cross-checking. After all, how would we know what the true nature of your poop was once you were taking creon? Seemed reasonable to daddy and me. *Let's see what she says*, I thought. I continued with it until I heard back.

In other baby news, you had successfully navigated your first vaccinations and development check with the GP. It felt good to have a normal appointment in amongst all the CF stuff!

'You're perfect,' he said to you after his examination.

I was getting other lovely comments from people, such as, 'He knows who his mummy is!' and 'He loves his mummy!' simply cos of how you looked at me. It made me worry that daddy might be feeling a bit left out, bonding-wise. I asked him that night, and he replied that he was a bit. Time to schedule more 'daddy time'.

Financially, The Butterfly Trust had suggested that we make detailed notes of how long everything was taking - from meds to physio to creon, including preparation and cleaning as well as the actual treatment. I was to note whether or not you sweated more than normal, resulting in more frequent clothes and bed changes (people with CF sometimes sweat more than others). I found this a bit difficult and really had to think about it, as I was just used to doing what I had to do.

However, it was very important for the benefits application. Luckily, they were going to act as advocates and help us with that whole process. There was no way our heads would have been able to cope with that on our own. I was desperate to be able to stay at home with you for as long as you needed me and, if benefits were going to help us afford to do that, then so be it. I didn't particularly like the idea of living on benefits, having worked for most of my adult life, but your needs and health were far more important than my pride.

The nurse got back about holding off on the creon. She said, 'Ok, if his poo changes then start the creon. Will get in touch Monday. Have a nice weekend.'

I felt a sense of relief. Almost how I imagine I'd feel if we heard they'd made a mistake and you didn't have CF. A small victory, I felt. The creon was one of the easier things on you, but I wanted to give your body the chance to do something for itself for as long as possible. You'd only get the one chance, cos if they were going to put you on it, you'd likely be on it for life.

I kept going over how well you slept and surely if you weren't getting enough nutrients, you'd be more narky and hungry and wake for a feed? I did still have a little bit of hope left in me. *I'm not giving up on this quite yet!* Later that day, your poop was green. *I suppose we'll know over the weekend if you're gonna need the creon or not, by your poop if nothing else.*

However, before long, instead of feeling comforted about your sleeping for long periods without waking for a feed, I started to stress. I worried that, without the creon, you might not be getting enough nutrients. So, I would wake you just to feed you. I planned on getting a poop sample from you after the weekend and take it to the GP myself. I felt like I didn't trust the nurse somehow. I knew it was my imagination (*it's not a conspiracy – he does have CF*), but still……I wanted to hand the sample in myself.

If he needs creon, then I can put the denial behind me, accept it and forget it. Get on with it and get on with our lives. Put the fear behind me!

I felt like I was worrying about anything and everything: it seemed never-ending; always thinking it must be related to CF; your poop; how often you peed; your breath; how much you ate……

In time, however, I soon came to realise that most things were baby-related, not CF-related, and gradually started to relax into motherhood.

Acceptance

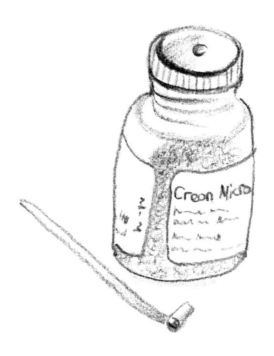

I dreamt that I was measuring out an exact amount of antibiotics for myself to take in front of you, to show you that I was doing it too.

PEP was still difficult. We kept trying different things, like doing it at different times of the day, in different locations, singing, whistling and using the mask on its own as a game before attaching the valve and resistor (the mask was fine, you didn't mind it, but when I added the other parts, there was lots of screaming, red face and tears). But I think I knew that it was just going to take time and no amount of singing, whistling, bouncing, moving about, silly daddy faces or baby Mozart was going to make much of a difference for a while. I tried to tell you that it'll get easier and you'll soon be old enough to understand what I'm saying, and why you have to do this. Difficult. On a lighter note, I'd been counting the minutes for PEP in my head, but when I switched to my small alarm clock with the second hand, I realised I'd been going too slow. *Wow, I can't even count to a minute anymore, ha.*

The nurse texted to arrange her next home visit, and I felt really annoyed. She'd only recently told us we'd play it by ear and she'd only come round if necessary! I texted back that we needed a break from all this medical stuff that we just wanted to do what we had to do and then forget about CF. She replied that they did need to see you between clinics. She was stressing me out. She never texted again that day. About a month later, it came to me that perhaps the nurse wanted to see you in between clinics to check that you were being looked after properly and that we were coping with it all. I guess it just takes your brain a while to come round to such realisations, especially when you just want left alone to get on with it.

I would find myself wondering about my body passing on the faulty gene to my baby; how could it *do that*? These thoughts were still not very far away, but were less frequent.

We had a bit of a breakthrough with PEP – yay! You cried on the first one but for the last four, yes four, you didn't! Daddy had *Minions* music on his phone and he was doing silly dances – you were fixated. So, he ordered the *Minions* DVD for you; I'd actually not seen it either, so we could sit and watch it together. I knew that tomorrow could be a different story again and if only it could be like that every time. Then you and I wouldn't hate (and dread) doing it. I could only hope that it did get easier.

About ten days later we got the news that you did, in fact, need the creon and we should restart it. They hadn't received your second poop sample result yet, but the pancreatic numbers of the first were so low that they didn't expect the second to show anything different. I felt a bit low again. Around this time, you were also bothered quite a bit by wind, which made you irritable and you cried a lot. I remember Google-ing 'CF and wind' but nothing came up; it was some relief to realise that it must just be a baby thing.

Every day and every night, we kept an eye on your nappies; as well as keeping a feeding diary, I continued to note how many wet nappies you had and how many poops you had done, while also noting their colour and checking for abnormal smells and textures - luckily, they always seemed normal enough to me. It's amazing how happy a person can be to see yellow or brown poop! The support worker from The Butterfly Trust had told us to keep an eye out for creon residue in your nappies too, as they could burn you.

Feeding now had to include a spoonful of fruit puree with a carefully calculated amount of creon added, dependent on how much of a feed you had. So, we bought a load of little tubs with lids, an ice tray and organic puree from the supermarket, then squeezed the whole sachet of puree into the tray and popped it into the freezer. Every night I'd take out one or two cubes of puree for the following day. My technique was to let you have one breast then I'd feed you the puree/creon before switching you to the other breast. That way, we made sure that you a) washed the creon down with milk, and b) had taken some food before giving you the creon. The amount of creon given was dependent on the amount of fat ingested, so it was a bit of a guessing game with breastfeeding, never quite knowing how much you would have at any given time. Your poop kept us right though, and I think we did a pretty good job. After your feed, I also checked your mouth – inside and around the outside – for any creon granules, making sure any present were removed; because they are technically digestive enzymes, they can burn. Likewise, I always checked my breasts to make sure none had been left there from your mouth. Giving you the creon halfway through the breastfeed helped ensure that the enzymes were ingested and not left in your mouth. You seemed to enjoy it, which made me smile and sigh with relief at the same time. *Aww, is that good? Is that one of the nicer things you have to take? Good.*

While it was extra tiring to have to concentrate on the delicate task of scooping out tiny granules from a small bottle with a fiddly little scoop, and tipping them one-handed onto a spoon of fruit puree (sometimes while half asleep), it did become quite routine a lot sooner than I had anticipated. I guess it's true what they say about the human spirit being highly adaptable and able to cope when it must. And this should give us all hope, whatever we're going through. I started to feel like I didn't have to worry about your poop quite as much, now that you were on the creon. Oh, by the way, those granules are like tiny ball bearings and a nightmare to tidy up if they're spilled. Luckily, that only happened once with me and it was bye-bye half a bottle of creon. I always made sure we had at least one spare bottle after that.

The rest of our routine was becoming well established now. I had a pretty tight system – a place for everything and everything in its place. I was particularly fussy about things like sterilising, hand washing, where I stored your meds, equipment and dummies, how I stored your syringes, using anti-bac hand gel when out in public places, having guests take their shoes off in the house, and so on. I was committed to keeping everything as hygienic as possible; I may have been a bit over-cautious, but as it was my gut feeling I went with it, as I always do. We got quite paranoid about being around anyone who was, or might be, coughing or sneezing. Even if I was due to take you to visit a friend or family member, it could be called off at the last minute if any one of us had even the hint of a sniffle. We did have to cancel quite a few plans, just to be on the safe side. For friends who didn't know about your condition, it was basic baby-safety: for everyone else, they completely understood. As time went on and you grew bigger and stronger, we relaxed a bit and so public outings and family gatherings became less of a worry. Of course, we still applied common sense, but the tight grip of fear diminished somewhat. I guess we were also growing in confidence with our knowledge of

CF. And we wanted you to live your life, experience things you should experience. Fall down, get hurt, pick yourself up, dust yourself off then do it all over again.

Another surprising 'intrusion' that came with CF, or a new diagnosis at least, was the amount of NHS mail that arrived through the letterbox. Hospital appointments, clinic updates, dietician formulas, breastfeeding/ creon charts to complete, physiotherapy routines, and so on. I hated seeing them. Every time another one came, my heart sank. *What now?* They were just reminders of something that I was still trying to forget. Then again, sometimes the letter was for a general baby appointment from the GP practice and I could unclench.

As for PEP, we had moved onto cheery nursery rhymes on YouTube, which you seemed to engage with so I pretty much relied on them every time now. Slowly, but surely, you started to relax and breathe gently into the mask without as much crying. Sometimes you didn't cry at all; not a peep! *Perhaps one day it'll always be like that.*

You had started laughing, such sweet, cute noises. Pure, total laughter. Made my heart laugh with you. Around this time I had the last physiotherapy session for my leg, which was great – one less thing to have to go to. My leg was slowly gaining mobility and strength; the pram had acted as a good crutch to lean on as I gained confidence walking again. I also started writing again, fiddling with existing stories I'd written. It was a welcome distraction, giving me something else to think about other than CF, which could only be a good thing. I had my last osteopath appointment as well; unfortunately I wasn't any wiser about the cause of the pain or the prognosis, but was getting referred via my GP for an x-ray and scan to help figure it out, so all was progressing there too. On the drive back from that last appointment, it was just you and me. We stopped on a lovely country road where I fed, changed and settled you back to sleep in your car seat. It was a beautiful sunny afternoon, and I met up with mum and one of my sisters for a coffee before heading for home. I felt like it had been a successful and happy day. For the first time, I really felt like the grief and pain was beginning to flow out of me, and I dared to believe that it would be getting easier from now on.

I dreamt that my mum nearly drowned. We were by a pool of water and needed to wash our boots. I tried, but realised it was too deep and came out and told mum not to go in. She went further over and tried, but she went right under. Her head bobbed up and down as she screamed, 'I can't swim!' It was cold. I was on the verge of jumping in after her, but woke myself up.

Our New Normal

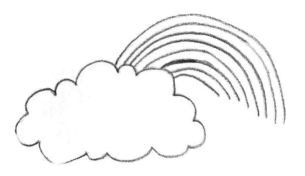

As the days passed, and we settled into our routines, we also started to realise that it wasn't so bad if we didn't think about it too much. That helped ease some of the fear and melodrama surrounding it, and we went back to seeing you - our beautiful little boy - as just you again. Ok, you happen to have a condition, but you're still you and most people have some shit or another to deal with in their lives. You aren't defined by CF and we refused to give it any more of our precious headspace than we already had. We would do what we had to do to keep you as healthy as possible, then we'd forget about it. I thought about what I'd say to you when you got a bit older, 'Yes, baby, you have CF, but take your meds, do your physio then get out there and enjoy your day.'

And that is what I do now. I give you your antibiotics, creon and vitamins, do your physio with you (once or twice a day depending on whether or not you have an infection), then we can forget about it. In fact, even as I'm doing meds and physio, I'm rarely thinking 'CF' anymore. 'It's just our new normal,' daddy says.

Through all the sadness and worry, I just had to look at your beautiful, happy face and I felt a smile spread across mine. In those moments, I knew that no matter what happened, everything was going to be alright.

I found out when Bookbug sessions were being held at the local library. Bookbug is run by the Scottish Book Trust, and is free. Babies, toddlers and pre-schoolers can enjoy singing nursery rhymes and reading stories with other children their age as well as the accompanying adults, with different sessions for different age groups. The sessions last about 30 minutes, and I had it in mind to take you along, even though I felt a bit anxious about the potential for coughs and sneezes amongst the other kids. I knew that the benefits of mingling would outweigh the risks, but I wouldn't be taking any chances – if you were under the weather, we wouldn't go and if anyone else was under the weather, we'd leave. On a sillier note, I was getting fed up washing my long hair and, as I once did in my early twenties, I put it in two ponytails then lopped half of it off.

Liberating!

Just doesn't matter.

It's only hair.

Not important.

The Butterfly Trust continued with our benefit applications until we were awarded the appropriate levels. We couldn't have done it without them; they were second to none. Also to thank with benefit advice and applications was our local Citizens Advice Bureau; you and I had numerous trips to their office. I will always fondly remember breastfeeding you as the advisor worked online to help us sort things out.

I don't know where we would have been without all these people guiding us and in such a timely manner. We have never been a particularly well-off family, so this assistance was invaluable in allowing us to afford even monthly basics. The Butterfly Trust also arranged a small grant to help us purchase a new washing machine and a dryer; up until this point we didn't have a dryer and had been informed that it wasn't a good idea to hang damp clothes in front of the fire anymore, as the dampness could exacerbate your condition. We were still learning so much, not least how wonderful charities such as these are to people in need; I guess you just don't appreciate such things until you find yourself in that situation. And it's only when you find yourself in that situation that you realise what you're actually capable of coping with. I would describe my relationship with CF at this point as being 'in limbo'. I'd accepted it, but I didn't want to talk about it.

I dreamt that someone I loved had CF and they were going to die before too long.

Following that dream, I felt a bit shaken again (some days, it didn't take much), and found myself Google-ing 'what does life-limiting mean?' The answer was along the lines of: illness or disease where it is expected that the person will die as a result. I'd initially believed it to mean that the person would be more limited in what they could do. The search made me wonder, again, about how long you'd live (always my main worry since diagnosis), and it bothered me that your body wasn't going to work 'properly', or as well as it should. Yes, it bothered me. But we had clinic the next day, and I figured that was probably why I was stressing like this, as clinic made me feel very uneasy (not to mention a bit trapped or controlled or something....?) We were going into the city after clinic for an unrelated appointment, and I felt it was important that we made that our routine – to have a coffee somewhere other than the hospital. I knew it would do me good to not just associate that city with CF.

That second clinic was a month and a half after the first one. We were told that they'd be approximately a month apart until everyone was happy with the routines, then they'd be every three months for the foreseeable future, eventually going to once a year. As it turned out, this clinic left me feeling a lot more positive than the first one. I think that had a lot to do with the fact that you didn't need any more medication – you were on everything you were going to be on, for now. Everyone was happy with you: your weight was good, you were following your centile well, they commented on your head control, your personality and your nice big thighs (the doctor liked to see nice big thighs on his CF patients!). As your head control was now much stronger, the physiotherapist added a new technique, called Autogenic Drainage, or AD, to apply in between the PEP mask. I basically squeezed your upper chest with my fingers, resisting the natural rise and fall, to encourage air to travel to the smaller airways in your lungs (improving ventilation); this helped to clear any mucus that might be stuck there.

Everyone was very positive, which was great. It all felt quite routine.

'CF is just part of who he is, not who he is,' the doctor very wisely reminded us.

By now, PEP was gradually becoming easier than it used to be, even with the added squeezes. We still sat on the bouncy ball, and varied the distraction viewing from nursery rhymes to *Despicable Me*. You still got antsy and would grab my hand holding the mask and try to get it off. You were strong! Still, I couldn't complain, it was a lot less stressful now and I was feeling a lot less daunted by it all.

One night I was out with the dog and you, asleep in your pram. I got to thinking about your condition and the future, which led me to life in general and what happens when we die. I thought about loved ones who'd passed away – human and animal – and what they may be doing. This then led to a weird thought: what if life is really just a game, a training ground before the 'real' life starts? What if life isn't the real life at all and when we die, we don't really die at all – we just decide we don't want to play anymore and we leave and go back home, to the real life. Who knows, but it started me rethinking everything, seeing the bigger picture which had more or less eluded me since your diagnosis. This life isn't necessarily the whole story; imagine all those we have lost, sitting somewhere else, telling their stories of how they stopped playing the game and returned home. Sounds crazy, I know. But really, who knows what happens when we die. And who knows when we will die. No-one. So, what's the harm in thinking out of the box and not taking our own struggles and issues so seriously? That's the conclusion I came to that evening anyway. In an 'a-ha!' moment, I saw that all of our problems weren't the most important thing in the world, that I don't know the truth of the universe and neither does anyone else (probably). Yes, things seem tough, but we will get through it and this world, this life, may not be all there is anyway – there may be somewhere better for us after all. Somewhere where none of this will even matter.

Yes, I was starting to regain some of my long-held faith in something greater than ourselves. Life, to me, seems meaningless without believing in something other than what we can see, touch, smell, taste or hear – something other than what we can prove. It's that *just knowing* belief that I had from childhood;

something is out there and that something is a good thing. It's going to be ok. Yes, there is joy, laughter and love in this world, but there is also incredible pain, suffering, struggle and heartache. And this world *without* something greater than all of that? For me, it just doesn't bear thinking about. The bible says that there remains faith, hope and love and that the greatest of these is love.

But.
For me?
The greatest of these is not love.
It's not even faith.
It is hope.

Get Busy Living

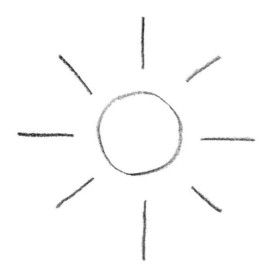

I dreamt about a fictional famous woman who had CF – she was in her 60's now. I thought it was very encouraging that someone with CF was that age.

You'd started communicating with squeaks and squeals (I think dolphins would have understood you better than I did!) and making a lot more eye contact. Adorable moments where you'd grab my hair and laugh joyfully; you loved it when I dangled my hair over your face. I felt a shift in my sensitivities now that I was a mother – so many things reminded me of you. Anytime I saw or read anything about a child, I immediately connected with the parents and felt a protective pull towards the child. Even if the child was an adult; daddy and I often watched documentaries about murder and such like, and when I saw the victim – or reconstruction of the victim – lying there, I'd think of you. Yes, I was seeing you in others: the boy being hurt, the man crying in despair, the disabled child, the frightened man. I saw the older men as my grown up you. Even girls and women in danger or pain, reminded me of you. I started to have frightening images of bad things happening to you and the adrenalin would rush through me. Things were resonating with me on an emotional level that pre-you would only have resonated on a logical level. Yes, I was becoming an ultra-sensitive, emotional wreck!

PEP with the AD squeezes was progressing well; you were doing so much better with less crying and struggling. We were all so impressed with you. Each session of physio had to end with the PEP mask, to make sure your lungs were cleared. You know, I was actually starting to enjoy your physio now, as I could see you were relaxing into it.

The CF Trust website was still a frightening prospect for me. Sometimes I had a glance at it, and immediately felt that it was a mistake. One minute you think there's hope and good news and the next it's all scary doom and gloom. That's why I didn't like to look. I'd 'liked' their Facebook page but wondered if I should 'unlike' it again, so I didn't keep getting updates that I might not want to see. Ignorance is bliss? For now anyway. Sigh.

I dreamt that you had died. Horrid. My lovely little baby boy. I couldn't accept it. In the dream, we were told that you could go at any time and we were making the most of you, but still......

That's what that website does to me. At times like that, I had to remind myself that none of us know how long we've got and to make the most of what we have. Perhaps that really is the answer.

I think what also helped was the fact that no-one needed to know you had a condition, and no-one would know to look at you. Daddy and I constantly found ourselves avoiding internet searches and reading the CF Trust newsletters; we just weren't ready for negative news. We only told immediate family about your diagnosis, and a very few close friends that we trusted. We felt it was your business who knew; that was your right and we didn't want to take that away from you before you were even old enough to speak. So, no posting it on Facebook for us. To be honest, I couldn't think of anything worse. Fast forward a year or so, and we were able to engage a lot more with the latest news, and there was a whole lot of it that was uplifting. What also helped was that our team at the hospital was very proactive and positive; we gradually learned to appreciate them and not hate them for giving us that dreadful news all those months ago. All credit to them for the wonderful work they do, and the manner in which they do it.

I spent a lot of time thinking about things I may say to you and ways in which I hope to help you see things a bit differently or more clearly. We hoped to raise you to see the bigger picture, to be grateful for life and every day; as we all should be. Once I had come to accept you had this condition, I started to understand that it wasn't so bad, and even on the days when I thought it was, there was still the silver lining of all the research being done and the race against time to be the company or person to discover the winning treatment or cure. That is one silver lining of having CF, I feel. The other silver lining for me, is the fact that you – and we – have been forced to face mortality. We have had the fact that we are all going to die shoved right into our faces, and guess what? We lived to tell the tale! It wasn't so bad to face that fact once we got over the shock. Really, how many people think about how short and precious life is, and that they won't always be here; that loved ones won't always be here? Sure, we don't want to dwell on it, obviously, but I sensed a shift in my perception of life and what may or may not come after (may, as I choose to believe). It is quite exciting really, and I no longer feel I'm sleepwalking through my days. I tend to appreciate you and every day we spend together a lot more than I have done with others; not just cos you are my baby, but cos I've had an electric shock of awareness shot through my soul. I want to keep awakening my mind to what really matters and take time to smell the roses, instead of the old, manic, 'rushing about' me.

I would hope we can pass that kind of outlook on to you. In an ironic way, I feel CF has given you – and us – the gifts of *life* and *time*. To be told you have a condition that may take you 'early' (but it won't, baby), encourages us all not to take a moment for granted and to be ready to face life head on. Think of it like this: instead of wasting any *time* sleepwalking, you can be full of awareness and full of the *life* you have been

118

given. As J.R.R Tolkien said, 'All we have to decide is what to do with the time that is given us.'

Imagine yourself as a teenager, knowing what you already know: how different may your attitude be to your peers? I hope you'll have lots of fun and be carefree, knowing that there's more to life than our physical body, and your mind is wild and free; life is a game, enjoy it! Live it to the fullest and live it long. One of my all-time favourite quotes from the excellent *Rita Hayworth and Shawshank Redemption* rings even more true now: 'It always comes down to just two choices. Get busy living or get busy dying.'

When I think about all the suffering in the world, human and animal, I don't know whether it's a way of coping with that pain or trying to alleviate it for those who suffer, but I imagine them when they die – particularly traumatic, painful deaths – having a laugh and exchanging stories with those already 'there' (wherever 'there' is, but I hope and pray that we go somewhere when we die, and meet again), about how they lived and died. 'You'll never guess what I had to go through,' or 'You'll never guess the horrible way I had to die!' In my image it's that training ground again.   The training ground for the life that comes after, the one that *is* real. It comforts me, and no-one can tell me for a fact that there isn't some truth in that, which comforts me further.

Sorry to mention the dreaded 'D' word again, but hey, we're not afraid of it anymore, right? I don't believe that dying is the end, and even if it was, you'll live loads before that happens. And remember, plenty of people die before they're 90 (or however long one expects to live). No-one knows how long they have to live, and that is the point! Appreciate every day you are alive, cos no-one is here forever and life, as they say, really is short for all of us. Everyone has something or another to put up with, and everyone dies. I know you'll have your down days but, whatever you go through, baby, we'll go through it together. And fear not, for I can assure you that your future is going to be filled with much wonder and possibility.

And who's to say that you won't be one of the future scientists who discovers a breakthrough treatment, or even better, a *cure* for cystic fibrosis? We hope there will be nothing to stop you from fulfilling whatever destiny or path that you choose.

Daddy and I had a meeting with a Genetic Counsellor, to discuss options if we were to have another baby. Even though we were still mentally and emotionally processing your diagnosis, we were keen on the idea of trying to give you a sibling. Obviously we would have to take the risk factor of being carriers of CF into account but, to be honest, by now we were pretty sure that the benefits of you having a sibling outweighed the risk (25%) of passing CF to another child. It was a lot to consider, but now that we knew how to better handle it all, it was nowhere near as daunting as it had been in the beginning.

You were taking your antibiotics and vitamins quite well now. There were still hiccups along the way, of course, but all-in-all it was becoming less of a stress for you, and therefore, me. As you were gaining weight, the dose was doubled which wasn't as frightening as it might have been. As long as it was for a good reason, such as weight gain, then we could accept that. You actually took it well, I felt so proud of you. The nurse told us that it would stay that dose for the foreseeable future, and she reminded us that you should be able to come off them altogether at three years old (only requiring them if you caught an infection).

I dreamt of babies last night. One of my sisters had you for some reason, and she wasn't letting me see you. She was doing things that I wouldn't do. It wasn't a pleasant dream. Later on that night, I dreamt of two kids - a boy and a girl. My other sister was there. At first I thought it was her kids, but soon realised they were mine. Again, my sister was not doing things with them that I would do. That wasn't a pleasant dream either.

Onwards and Upwards

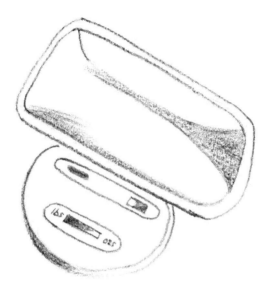

It is very important for people with cystic fibrosis to stay as active as possible, as this helps clear the mucus from their lungs and keeps them physically fitter and stronger. Obviously this is limited for a baby, but at clinic they offered a variety of suggestions which were relevant to your age, such as bouncing on the birthing ball or a small trampoline, swimming and tummy time, eventually leading to crawling, singing, walking, dancing and so on. They would assist us by encouraging you at the different stages of your development, if needed. Basically, as you grew up, it was important for you to try as many different physical activities as possible, to find which you were most interested in pursuing and to keep at it. So, as well as PEP/AD, exercise would effectively become part of your daily physio. As you grew into a toddler, you enjoyed learning to walk, particularly out in nature with our dog. By the age of two, you barely wanted in your pram anymore and could happily walk, run and explore for several miles or sit for a while in your push-along trike.

When you were five months old, the dietician came to visit us at home to discuss weaning. She had some helpful charts explaining which foods needed creon and which didn't, some recipe ideas and general nutrition information relating to your age. We were to add the creon to food containing fat, protein or carbohydrate and I was relieved to hear that there were actually foods that *didn't* require creon, such as most fruit and veg (except avocado, which is exceptionally high in fat). We were to add it in relation to the fat content, using the following calculation to measure how much:

1-2g fat = ¼ scoop
3-4g fat = ½ scoop
5-6g fat = ¾ scoop
7-8g fat = 1 scoop

We would start off with that dose and see how it went, adjusting it if need be as time went on.

When I first received all this info, I felt overwhelmed; I did not want you to need this stuff and I was useless at maths. I felt it was all so much more to cope with and it made me feel a bit down again. I knew if this had been for a pet cat or dog I'd have been delighted the vet had something that I could give to help the digestion of food and, in return, their general wellbeing. So I couldn't understand why I was struggling so much with the concept of you having to take this. Didn't I want what was best for you? Deep down though, I knew I was just resisting the fact that you needed all of this crap, and how I wished that you didn't. *I hope I get there. I'm sure I will.* After all, I'd more or less accepted the antibiotics and vitamins. PEP was still hard for both of us. *When it's easier for him, it'll be easier for me.*

At least it was the last thing we had to do, the last piece of this nightmare puzzle. No more surprises, no more meds. And I figured we could be left alone to get on with our lives now, apart from clinic appointments, etc. We could get our lives back and not have to put up with all these infernal home visits. At first, I wasn't 100% convinced that you needed it. Eventually, I gradually started to accept it and also gained more trust in our team. *They're not out to get us or to make our life hell: they're just telling it like it is and one day we'll appreciate that.* But these realisations only come with time.

At six months old we started the weaning process, which was a lot of fun. You had a hearty appetite. The dietician and health visitor were on hand for advice, as and when needed, and you had regular weight checks. I found adding the creon a bit of a challenge at first but practice makes perfect, as they say. I eventually got so used to adding creon to your food, that I sometimes had to stop myself adding it to mine as well; it all just became second nature to me and I barely thought anything of it. I even got to grips with the various calculations without much effort. There were other things to take into account though, such as if you'd been given your creon dose for a particular meal but you didn't eat it all (which became more and more common as you grew into a fussy toddler!), we would have to top up your fat content to match the dose with something like cheese, peanut butter or yogurt – something that contained fat and was easy to add the creon granules to. Alternatively, if you'd eaten something containing fat but hadn't had the enzymes yet, we had to make sure we added them within about five to ten minutes for them to do their job. Fresh raspberries were really good for dropping creon into in an emergency! We just had to ensure there were no creon granules left in your mouth after eating; a glug of milk, water or juice washed them down. I grew less stressed if you had an infection and were on double meds and physio, seeing it as something you needed without thinking too much about why. *Do it, then let's get on with our day,* became my inner mantra.

Around this time, we took you for your first swim in the public pool. It was a bit scary for us as we felt you were very vulnerable to potential infections, especially being half naked in a swimming pool, but the benefits had to outweigh that risk. We put you in your large, inflatable swim ring and swirled you around in the warm water; you were mesmerised. We stayed in half an hour and vowed to go back regularly to get you used to it, as swimming would become a staple form of exercise for you.

Clinics were running more smoothly now, and we found it much less of a stress. Going to the hospital, while still making me feel a bit numb until we got out again, wasn't as daunting as it had previously been. We were getting into the routine, and now knew more or less what to expect. Most clinics did last between two to three hours, which was quite tiring for us all, but we usually came out with plenty of positivity and even a bit of laughter (it *is* the best medicine, after all). The team were extremely happy with your progress, and you were thriving along your growth centiles.

We felt so grateful for the NHS and free prescriptions; abidec alone can cost anything from £4 - £6 and goodness knows how much the antibiotics and creon are, let alone the PEP equipment and whatever else you may need in the future. I worried about future drugs not being available on the NHS; would they be available privately? *We can worry about that later.*

I was starting to think along the lines of practising yoga, meditation and deep breathing with you when you were old enough. These were things I was already into, so I hoped to pass that on to you. Yoga would be excellent for relaxing, stretching your muscles (with particular interest in your chest area), and conscious breathing, while meditation and deep breathing would exercise your lungs as well as relax you. It was my hope that these techniques would be especially useful to you in times of stress and worry.

Family and social days out took some planning. Along with the usual baby-related paraphernalia, we also had to make sure we had enough creon, puree, antibiotics and syringes (if we were staying late), cool bag and ice for puree and meds, and your PEP mask if you had an infection and were on physio twice a day. If we'd had to leave before we'd had time to do even your normal once-a-day physio, we took your PEP equipment with us to do it during the day; this often meant also taking the iPad with us for your nursery rhymes during physio. Not everyone knew about your condition, so there was a level of secrecy involved with administering meds and physio. That could make things a bit tricky, logistically, but we always found a way. Maintaining your confidentiality has been a very high priority from the moment you were diagnosed. All that said, we had some pretty special days out in your first year of life and most of the time you came home without catching anything off anyone. This gave us some confidence that you were more robust than we'd anticipated, and this was a very positive realisation going forward.

Clinic appointments were now every three months, as we'd settled into a routine with your treatment and everyone was happy with your progress. The nurse still came out to our house at regular intervals in between clinic to do routine cough swabs. If you'd picked up an infection, or we suspected you might have, she would do a nasal brush (if you had a runny nose) as well as a cough swab – needless to say you didn't enjoy either – to ascertain which antibiotic to treat it with, alongside your regular prophylactic daily dose. I was now able to see the nurse and the rest of the team as more of the support network that they were, rather than our enemies. As winter approached, you had your flu jab at the GP practice.

By the time your first Christmas approached, things were running very smoothly indeed. We'd settled well into your treatment regime and you were tolerating everything so much better as you grew bigger and stronger. CF had taken a back seat in our consciousness - *why ruin today's pleasures by worrying about the future?* - and I'm pleased to say that we were far more interested in your amazing developmental achievements in the past months. You were almost one year old and had given us so much joy already, not to mention how much we'd learned from you. Every day was a new experience and there was not a day went by that you didn't make us smile, laugh, burst with love. You were sociable and charming from the get-go and made everyone's day. I get the feeling that you're always going to have that light-hearted, fun, charming nature. I pray that you hold onto your beautiful light, your beautiful spirit, your bravery and strength. We will always burst with love for you, baby.

The Future is Bright

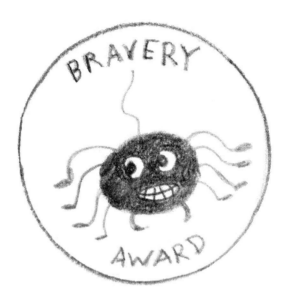

Yes, as I watched you grow through your first year, I was amazed at how much it meant to me to be with you and to experience each milestone with you. Your first giggle, first babble, first tooth, first tentative crawl – I knew it would all mean something to me, but the joy, delight and love was something I couldn't have known before you. As I watched you play, squeak and smile, my heart filled with happiness and love and I smiled inside and out. *I will protect and love you always.* I was a very thankful mummy indeed.

We planned a little party of family and a few friends for your first birthday. Just a small gathering at our house, nothing over-the-top as that just isn't our style. By that time, we were pretty much settled into our life with CF, and didn't feel anywhere near as overwhelmed and anxious as we had all those months ago. Things seemed to be running smoothly enough and the fear of people visiting, or us visiting other people, had diminished quite a bit. Sure, we still took sensible precautions and sure, we still had to juggle meds, physio and keep you away from 'coughers and sneezers' (sometimes doing all those things in secret, when around people who didn't know about your condition), but even all that was second nature by now. We couldn't believe it was already a year since you were born. So fast, yet so crammed with devastation, anger, guilt, depression, anxiety, fear, love, joy, gratitude, laughter, strength and amazement.

All-in-all, that second winter came and went without you catching too many bugs. Not long after you'd turned one year old, and almost a year to the day you were diagnosed, you had your first annual review. If you remember, on our first visit to the hospital after your diagnosis, you had bloods taken and not long after that, you had your first scan and x-ray The annual review was a follow up on those procedures and would take place every year as close to your birthday as possible. Prior to your appointment, the nurse had made a home visit to explain what would happen at the review and that they didn't expect any changes to be needed, but if anything it would be to adjust your vitamins.

The review basically consisted of an early start to travel to the hospital for an ultrasound scan of your abdomen and pelvis, followed by a chest x-ray and finally blood tests. The nurse explained that they like to get their CF patients in for scans and x-rays first to minimise infection risks, hence the early appointments. You wriggled and cried your way through both x-ray and scan, even with daddy or I by your side soothing you. Not surprising, seeing as you were only a year old: how do you explain to a one year old to lie still while they look at your insides with the big machinery? We felt tense and a bit anxious; we knew how important today was for measuring future x-rays and scans against, but we were very glad for you when they were finally over. The doctor reassured us that everything in the scan looked normal as far as she could tell, which helped us relax a little (quite hard to relax in the clinical environment with your baby agitated and sobbing). I wiped off the scan gel, changed your nappy and sorted your clothes. Not forgetting your dummy and comfort blanket! Warm, dry and happy again. We headed to children's outpatients for the blood test, which I was especially dreading.

Once again, we were pleasantly surprised with how well it went. The nurse, who we hadn't met before, was exceptional. While I held you on my knee, daddy and the nurse distracted you and you were so good when the needle went into your arm (thank goodness not your hand this time). It didn't take long at all and the nurse brought you a small toy piano still in its packaging, which she told us was left over from their Christmas gift stock. You also got a couple of bravery stickers. Very brave indeed. I will treasure that wee piano and those stickers forever. All done, we breathed a big sigh of relief and headed to Dobbies.

Unfortunately, being born in the winter, your annual reviews were going to fall at a time of year when you might not be in 100% health and for the first two, you weren't. I worried that this could potentially show false results, especially in your chest x-rays, but our team doctor assured us that this is all taken into account and not to worry about it. Turns out that you had developed bronchiolitis around the time of this first annual review. You were prescribed extra antibiotics (to treat secondary bacterial infection), physio twice a day, plenty of rest and fluids. You were over it completely within a few weeks and back to full strength. Apparently you'd done very well, as some babies, even those without CF or other medical conditions, can be hospitalised. I felt proud of you and it brought me a sense of relief to know that, even something potentially that bad, can pass by without too much intervention. Perhaps this CF lark wasn't going to be such a nightmare after all. Long may your body be strong and healthy enough to fight this every step of the way. *Remember, whatever you go through, baby, we'll go through it together.*

We got a letter with the results of the annual review, followed by a more in-depth discussion at your next clinic appointment. We were happy we'd got that first one out of the way and, as many things with CF were now turning out, it wasn't half as bad as we'd anticipated. At least we now knew what to expect, and were relieved to learn that neither the scan, bloods nor x-ray showed up anything abnormal. The team were delighted with your progress developmentally, and, as usual, you charmed your way through clinic appointments, which helped mummy and daddy forget why we were actually there.

Now that you were no longer breastfeeding, we could plan your antibiotic doses to be given on an empty stomach, which was the best way to administer them; something we'd been unable to do with breastfeeding, as we never knew exactly when you'd feed. This meant our morning routine became something like this: wake up, give your morning antibiotic, let you play with your toys for an hour, physio then breakfast with vitamins and creon. Your evening antibiotic would be given two hours after your supper, more often than not, once you'd gone to bed. So, one hour before food or two hours after = on an empty stomach. This routine worked very well for us and we could adapt it if needed. We made every effort to allow you to get the most from the medication and hopefully at three years old you'd be taken off the antibiotics, only being given them if you had an infection.

So, things settled into: daily meds and physio, three-monthly clinics, home visits in between for routine cough swabs, swimming fun, vaccinations, long walks in the fresh air, double antibiotics and physio whenever you caught an infection, Bookbug at the library, annual reviews at the hospital. Daddy and I kept one eye on the CF Trust newsletters, but kept the other one shut; we were accepting of you having CF but were still wary of too much information, or anything negative that we did not want to be focussing on – not when there were so many positive steps happening now and in the pipeline.

At one and a half years old, we took you on your first holiday, thanks to family support and The Butterfly Trust, who arranged for a donation to be made for a respite break for us. As we'd already planned to stay in the UK until you were at least three (to tie in with your 'big' review at the clinic, when we hoped you could come off the prophylactic antibiotics), this was perfect for us. We had the most glorious ten days in the sun – yes, the sun (we got lucky with the weather!) – and it really was the most relaxing ten days we'd all had since you were born. You were growing more and more fascinated by nature and wildlife, just like mummy and daddy; we enjoyed loads of outdoor fun and fresh air. Of course, we were vigilant about hygiene and infection risks and continued with your meds and physio routine as usual, but other than that, CF could not have been further from our minds. Many, many thanks to the family members and The Butterfly Trust for their kind donations; we simply were not in the position to have considered such a lengthy break without it.

While you had settled well into the PEP mask – barely acknowledging it was on your face at all now – AD squeezes started getting difficult for me as you were getting bigger; I was finding it hard to stretch my hands around your growing chest. The physiotherapist mentioned that we could soon start introducing blowing games, such as using straws to blow bubbles into water, juice and particularly milk, which made nice big, fun bubbles apparently. I made a mental note to add straws to my next online shopping list. In the meantime, we could try toys designed for blowing into. I started searching online, and found a whistle that sounded like a train horn, bath whistles (that you fill with water and they make different notes) and a variety of other musical instrument toys. We also decided to add a new trampoline to your Christmas list, encouraged by the physiotherapist, as your old one was getting a bit weathered. Outdoor play and adventures (which you were getting a lot of, being part of an outdoorsy family) carried a few extra risks that we had to bear in mind. A common bacterium called pseudomonas aeruginosa, which is found in soil and stagnant water, can cause chest infections in those with compromised lungs. Moist leaves/foliage (mould), mud, wet sand and stagnant puddles were all things that we had to be wary of. We didn't necessarily have to avoid them altogether (try keeping an energetic toddler out of muddy puddles!), but it was imperative that we thoroughly washed your hands after coming into contact with any of these. Alternatively, we could use anti-bac hand gel when out and about. Some people might put gloves on their child, but we opted for hand washing and gel. We wanted to protect you, but at the same time we didn't want to 'over-protect' you or limit your outdoor experiences. You have to live your life, just like anyone else does. Go ahead and enjoy everything you want to enjoy, baby! Sure, there may be things you struggle to do, or cannot do, but that could happen to anyone. Let go of the things you feel unable to do, then take one step at a time into your happiness and go for it! Do not be afraid, do not let this hold you back. Be brave and strong and careful, but do not let this hold you back. We want your childhood to be filled with love, laughter and fun, and we hope that you carry that with you into adulthood.

While you were blossoming, I did still have a few inner panics about your fussy feeding phases, freaking out that you'd need a feeding tube if you didn't eat enough (you needed a constant high fat, high calorie diet). The nurse reassured me that you were nowhere near that stage, and there were many things they could try before it ever got to that, if necessary. At clinic, the doctor always assured us that your feeding habits were entirely age-appropriate and nothing to do with CF. I did wonder if the daily antibiotics were depressing your appetite, though no-one had mentioned that possibility. I probably wouldn't have been anywhere near as anxious if you didn't have a health condition, but gradually managed to calm down and see the bigger picture. You were eating a healthy, balanced diet over the course of a week – some days you'd eat more, some days you'd eat less – and you were gaining weight and looking great. Yes, I was still learning the art of chilling out when it came to you-related stuff.

Before you were two years old, you'd pretty much stopped having afternoon naps, unless you fell asleep in the car on the way back from a long walk or day out. It almost seemed like you were just too damn busy enjoying your life for naps, cramming as much into a day as possible. You'd sleep at bedtime like any other busy person! It's funny, I used to try and imagine what my son would look like, but I never expected him to be as beautiful and vibrant as you. You amaze me every day. I find myself fixated by you on a regular basis. I could just sit and stare at you in wonderment all day long, which seemed to be the reaction of most people who met you. You are a perfect little soul.

Just before your second birthday, I started writing down my dreams again, with the aim of learning how to lucid dream (to be aware that you're dreaming and to interact with your unconscious mind within the dream). I'd started about a year before but my dream journal got left in the drawer for several months as I continued with everyday life. This time round, I had high hopes that I'd succeed as others have, and that the practice would reap great rewards. One of my main hopes was to one day encourage you to keep doing it (apparently all children lucid dream naturally, whether we're aware of it as children though, I'm not sure) and, who knows, once you could do it, you might be able to strengthen your lungs or do some physio within your dreams. According to what I'd read, the mind can't tell the difference between what's real and what's 'imagined' or dreamt, and so the physiological benefits are the same for both. Quite astounding really, and very exciting if that's true! Many people had reportedly achieved great things when they woke up from practising within their dreaming mind. I strongly believed if there was one special thing I could teach you, it would be this. That is how much faith I had – and still have – in lucid dreaming. Sure, it was going to take some time to master, but I was determined to do it.

Shortly after you turned two years old, we attended your second annual review at the hospital. Although you started out calm and trusting, casually eating your tub of chopped fruit, we ended up with a repeat of the previous year: you squirming and screaming your way through the x-ray and scan. You took the blood test a bit better, this year with a video on the big screen for distraction. As with the year before, we felt guilt at having to put you through all this. However – and I feel that this is a big 'however', considering the circumstances – that guilt was nowhere near as potent as the previous year, as we were now armed with much more perspective, knowledge, experience and a year's worth of wonderful memories of our happy, relaxed, adaptable son. I knew that you

144

could handle this; that you could handle anything. Results of the second annual review were great; nothing at all to worry about at this point. You were well nourished and your x-ray and scan showed nothing abnormal or unexpected.

When you were first diagnosed, the doctor, who is actively involved in international conferences with other specialists in the field, said to us that there had never been a better time to have CF. As strange as that may sound, it is true: research has never been so advanced, treatment has never been so targeted, people are living healthier lives and for longer. At the time of writing this book, to quote the CF Trust website:

'We're on the cusp of something momentous. Developments in genetic science like gene editing and gene therapy are offering us long-term hope for beating cystic fibrosis. At the same time we are investing in cutting-edge stem cell research, and exploring the potential of health technology. Currently, we are experiencing the most exciting period in the history of cystic fibrosis research. Over the next few years we expect research into transformational treatments will bring about a revolution for people with the condition.'

Research into life expectancy and predicted survival has revealed that mortality rates have been dropping year on year. If that trend continues then the survival age of those diagnosed at birth will continue to improve.

Drugs to break down mucus in people with CF (and therefore reduce lung damage) are being tested for their efficacy. As I write, the fight to ensure that all these new drugs are available on the NHS, for all who need them, continues.

All-in-all, as a family, we are feeling positive and hopeful about the future. About *your* future.

A Letter from Mummy and Daddy

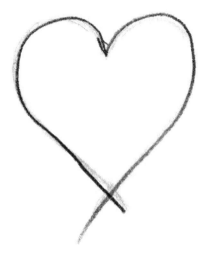

Our precious, beautiful, splendiferous baby boy,

Mummy wanted to tell your story - our story - for three reasons. One, was as a gift to you when you grow up, to open up a part of mummy and daddy to you; to show you how it all started as you obviously won't remember any of this. Two, was in the hope that other parents and carers of newly diagnosed children would read our story and feel confidence that it really *does* get easier, and they really *can* cope. And three, to try and raise awareness and money for two very worthy and important charities: the Cystic Fibrosis Trust and The Butterfly Trust. We hope our story can help all of you, in those individual ways.

Of course we worry about the future, we worry about life expectancy and how your health will be as you grow up. But it doesn't make sense to focus on that if it means we're missing out on *today*. And today is good. You've been keeping so well since diagnosis, and none of it is as daunting as we'd thought it would be. We've read of other babies and toddlers needing more meds, physio and hospital stays so we're not sure if they have a different variation of CF or if we've just been lucky so far – whatever the reason, long may it continue. Let's put our faith in the scientists and research companies who are working hard on treatments, treatments that will make a massive positive impact on the health of CF patients like never before. In the meantime, we have lofty plans for holidays we'd like to take you on, such as Lapland and swimming with dolphins. We'll do our very best to enable you to experience such wonders; open up the world to you at a young age. It may involve a credit card or two, but it'll definitely be worth that! You gotta dream big, little one.

'Don't sweat the small stuff,' they say. Ok, CF isn't small stuff but we get the feeling that you're not gonna sweat it anyway. We're not all that concerned about how you'll deal with your condition as you grow up, cos you seem to have this spirit about you: a glowing, fighting spirit that gives the impression you're gonna be far too busy enjoying your life to worry about stuff like that. Sure, there'll be tough days, but who doesn't have tough days? That's the attitude we hope to pass on to you, but to be honest, we think it's you that has passed it onto us – before you were even two years old. Don't ever lose that joy, baby.

Yes, cystic fibrosis is bad, but - you? You are so very, very good, our little friend. In every possible sense of the word.

Mummy and daddy don't know what the future holds. All we have, and all we know, is the here and now and right now you are thriving. Let us tell you, that puts a huge smile on our faces; it gives us great hope and optimism for the future. We really do have every faith in the wonderful scientists who are working towards better treatments and a cure. If you needed one of our lungs, we would give it, but it won't come to that. Every night after reading your bedtime stories, singing your rhymes and listening to daddy strum his guitar, mummy whispers in your ear that she loves you then prays that you live a long and healthy life.

You are our loving, sweet, funny, charming, clever, entertaining, beautiful son who is the light of our life. Everyone who meets you falls in love with you at first sight, then falls deeper with your cheeky grin. Our hearts burst with love and pride when we are near you; your soul sings brightly, loud and clear. You are vivid and luminous, full of loving energy and light. Obviously, if we could take CF away from you, we would, but we cannot. Hopefully scientific research can. But, in any case, our little friend, our little splendour, please know this: there is absolutely nothing we would change about you. Yes, you – our precious star - have a life-limiting condition and, yes, things may get difficult from time to time. Yes, we are having to do things we never anticipated we'd have to do, and things we wish you didn't have to go through. Yes, raising you has changed from what we'd expected, but....that's ok.

It's just our new normal.

with all our love,
mummy and daddy
xxxx

'You are made of kindness and possibility and brilliance. Everything you are made of, the stars are made of.And though the stars shine only at night, when it is dark, your light shines always.'

- The Man Made of Stars
M.H Clark

Acknowledgements

Special thanks to your aunties and granny (daddy's mum) for proofreading, editing and formatting; daddy for helping with the graphics and cover layout; family and friends for all their love, support and positivity; daddy's folks for their unbelievably kind financial help; our team at the hospital; The Butterfly Trust for all their support and assistance; the Cystic Fibrosis Trust for all their hard work, research and providing a light at the end of the tunnel and, of course, you! You are our inspiration and you give us strength and hope that we have never known before. Here's to the future, baby. Let's enjoy our game of life together!

All proceeds from the sale of this book will be donated equally between the Cystic Fibrosis Trust and The Butterfly Trust.

The author's name has been changed to protect identities. She lives in Scotland with her family. If you would like to contact her, you can do so at: graceymac@yahoo.com

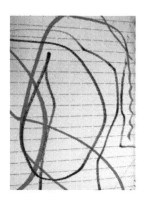

artwork by you, baby © 2018

References/Resources

www.cysticfibrosis.org.uk
www.butterflytrust.org.uk
www.nhs.uk
www.scottishbooktrust.com
www.citizensadvice.org.uk
www.charliemorley.com

The Lord of the Rings, J.R.R Tolkien,
Rita Hayworth and Shawshank Redemption,
Stephen King
The Man Made of Stars, M.H Clark

Printed in Great Britain
by Amazon